OSTEOPOROSIS

OSTEOPOROSIS
PATHOGENESIS AND MANAGEMENT

Editor

R. M. FRANCIS
MB, ChB, MRCP

Honorary Consultant Physician
Senior Lecturer in Medicine (Geriatrics)
Department of Medicine (Geriatrics)
University of Newcastle upon Tyne
Newcastle General Hospital
Newcastle upon Tyne
NE4 6BE, UK

Consultant Editor

W. CARSON DICK

KLUWER ACADEMIC PUBLISHERS
DORDRECHT / BOSTON / LONDON

Distributors

for the United States and Canada: Kluwer Academic Publishers, PO Box 358, Accord Station, Hingham, MA 02018–0358, USA
for all other countries: Kluwer Academic Publishers Group, Distribution Center, PO Box 322, 3300 AH Dordrecht, The Netherlands

British Library Cataloguing in Publication Data

Osteoporosis
  1. Man. Bones. Osteoporosis
  I. Francis, R. M.

  616.7'1
  ISBN 0–7462–0086–2

Library of Congress Cataloguing-in-Publication Data

Osteoporosis / editor, R. M. Francis.
      p.   cm.
    Includes bibliographical references.
    ISBN 0–7462–0086–2 : U.S. : £30.00 (U.K. : est.)
    1. Osteoporosis.   I. Francis, R. M. (Roger Michael)
    [DNLM: 1. Osteoporosis.   WE 250 08513]
  RC931.073076   1990
  616.7'16—dc20
  DNLM/DLC
  for Library of Congress   89–20123
                                                                 CIP

Copyright

Published in the United Kingdom by Kluwer Academic Publishers, PO Box 55, Lancaster, UK.

Kluwer Academic Publishers BV incorporates the publishing programmes of D. Reidel, Martinus Nijhoff, Dr W. Junk and MTP Press.

Printed in Great Britain by Butler & Tanner Ltd, Frome and London

CONTENTS

LIST OF AUTHORS

I. P. Braidman
Department of Medicine
(Endocrinology)
University of Manchester
Clinical Sciences Building
Hope Hospital, Eccles Old
Road
Salford M6 8HD
UK

C. Cooper
Rheumatology Unit
Bristol Royal Infirmary
Bristol BS2 8HW
UK
and
MRC Environmental
Epidemiology Unit
Southampton General Hospital
Southampton SO9 4XY
UK

C. E. Davison
Department of Medicine
(Geriatrics)
University of Newcastle upon
Tyne
Newcastle General Hospital
Newcastle upon Tyne NE4 6BE
UK

R. M. Francis
Department of Medicine
(Geriatrics)
University of Newcastle upon
Tyne
Newcastle General Hospital
Newcastle upon Tyne NE4 6BE
UK

D. M. Reid
Department of Rheumatology
City Hospital
Urquhart Road
Aberdeen AB9 8AU
UK

A. Rodgers
Department of Medicine
(Geriatrics)
University of Newcastle upon
Tyne
Newcastle General Hospital
Newcastle upon Tyne NE4 6BE
UK

P. L. Selby
Department of Medicine
University of Newcastle upon
Tyne
Framlington Place
Newcastle upon Tyne NE4 6BE
UK

PREFACE

Osteoporosis is one of the most important diseases facing the ageing population because of the high prevalence of fractures, the enormous costs in health care funds required to deal with the consequence of these fractures, and the substantial effect in terms of suffering and disability. One-third of women over age 65 will have vertebral fractures, and the life-time risk of hip fracture in white women (15%) is as great as that of breast, endometrial, and ovarian cancer combined. The life-time risk of hip fracture in men (5%) is as great as the risk of prostate cancer. Hip fracture is fatal in up to 20% of cases. One-half of survivors are unable to walk unassisted and 25% are confined to long-term care in nursing homes. The recent awareness that osteoporosis is a treatable and partly preventable disease of the elderly, and not just the inevitable consequence of ageing, comes at a time of rapid progress in measurement of bone mass and in a better understanding of the physiology and pathophysiology of bone cell function.

Thus, this new book by Dr R. M. Francis and his colleagues on osteoporosis is particularly timely. Because it contains only six chapters, it is of manageable length. Although the book is multi-authored, it is well balanced and bears the imprint of Doctor Francis who is a world-recognized authority in this area. Chapter 1, 'Bone Mass Throughout Life: Bone Growth and Involution', is written by Dr C. Cooper and reviews patterns of bone loss and fractures throughout life from both the pathophysiological and epidemiological perspective. The relationship between bone loss and fracture is discussed in detail and the use of bone densitometry in diagnosis of established disease and its potential use in assessing future risk for osteoporosis are carefully reviewed. Chapter 2, 'Cellular Mechanisms of Bone Resorption and Formation', is written by Dr I. P. Braidman and covers bone cell physiology, bone remodelling, and mechanisms of control by systemic hormonal and by local growth factors. This chapter brings the reader up to date on the enormous advances made in this area during the last five years. Chapter 3, 'The Pathogenesis of Osteoporosis', is written by Dr R. M. Francis and stresses the multifactorial nature of the disease together with a lucid review of the interaction of the various causal factors. Chapter 4, 'Oestrogen and Bone' is written by Dr P. L. Selby and focuses on the effect of oestrogen on bone and the consequences of oestrogen deficiency on the skeleton. It is appropriate to give a full chapter to this because of the important role that the menopause plays in pathogenesis. The recent demonstration that bone cells contain oestrogen and androgen receptors provides a rationale for the effect of sex steroid deficiency in producing bone loss and indicates that bone cells fulfil the criteria of a target tissue for sex steroid action. Chapter 5, 'Corticosteroid Osteoporosis', is written by Dr D. M. Reid and focuses on the main cause of secondary osteoporosis encountered in clinical practice, particularly in rheumatological practice. The final chapter, 'The Management of Osteoporosis', is written by Doctor Francis and colleagues and provides a careful review of the diagnostic workup and approaches to prevention and treatment.

This useful book covers the major aspects of osteoporosis in an easily accessible form. It fills the niche between review articles and chapters in medical and sub-specialty textbooks which provide inadequate detail and the large comprehensive textbooks which are targeted mainly at the specialist and the research scientist. It should be particularly valuable to practising clinicians, house staff and medical students who wish to know more about the causes of osteoporosis, its diagnosis, and its management.

B. Lawrence Riggs, MD
Consultant, Division of
Endocrinology and Metabolism
Purvis and Roberta Tabor
Professor of Medical Research
Mayo Medical School
Rochester, MN 55905, USA

1

BONE MASS THROUGHOUT LIFE: BONE GROWTH AND INVOLUTION

C. COOPER

Osteoporosis, defined as a reduction in bone mass[1], constitutes a major public health problem. This stems from its association with fractures of the hip, vertebrae and distal radius. This chapter reviews current concepts of bone structure, the methods for measuring bone mass, the patterns of change in bone mass with ageing and the relationship between bone mass and fracture risk.

BONE STRUCTURE

The human skeleton consists of two types of bone: cortical and trabecular[2]. Cortical bone is the compact layer which predominates in the shafts of long bones. Trabecular bone is composed of a series of thin plates which form the interior meshwork of bones, particularly the vertebrae, pelvis and ends of long bones. Overall, the adult skeleton is about 80% cortical and 20% trabecular bone[3]. Both cortex and trabeculae contribute to bone strength, and each bone has its own normal proportion of cortical and trabecular components[4,5]. The shafts of long bones, such as the radius and ulna, are at least 90% cortical, whereas vertebrae are mostly composed of trabecular bone[5,6]. Trabecular bone, with its greater surface area, is metabolically more active than cortical bone and therefore more responsive to influences which alter mineral homeostasis. Conditions which predispose to rapid bone loss, such as oestrogen deficiency, thus tend to affect trabecular bone more quickly than cortical bone[3].

Bone mineral

The specific feature distinguishing bone from all other tissues except dentine is the presence of bone mineral. This is a calcium phosphate complex with the overall composition of hydroxyapatite. Although initially present in amorphous form, this soon becomes crystalline. Mineral is deposited on the collagenous matrix to which it adds structural rigidity, as well as providing a reservoir for 99% of body calcium. The chemical and cellular processes controlling mineralization are not clearly understood. The concentrations of calcium and phosphate in extracellular fluid are sufficient to maintain crystallization, and it may be that this is normally prevented by inhibitors such as pyrophosphate. The alkaline phosphatase released by active osteoblasts might then promote mineralization by degrading these inhibitor molecules. The laying down of early bone crystals appears to be enhanced by matrix vesicles, which are derived from chondrocytes and osteoblasts. Although these vesicles have been shown to play a part in the mineralization of trabecular bone, this has not been demonstrated for cortical bone.

Bone collagen

The organic matrix of bone is 90% collagen. The remaining 10% comprises various bone proteins such as osteocalcin, sialoprotein, proteoglycans and osteonectin. Collagen is the main extracellular body protein, and about half of it is found in bone. Collagen comprises a family of molecules sharing a repetitive triple-helical configuration. It is synthesized by the fibroblast or osteoblast from long polypeptides, or alpha chains, three of which constitute each collagen molecule. There are at least ten genetically different collagens, with specific tissue distributions and properties suited to their functions. For example, basement membrane collagen is loosely organized, while collagen fibres in bone are tightly packed. Normal adult bone collagen is

2

deposited in layers of parallel fibres of uniform diameter and its anatomy reflects the rate at which it is synthesized[7]. When skeletal synthesis is markedly accelerated, such as accompanying a fracture or hyperparathyroidism, the collagen assumes a woven pattern with variably sized, randomly arranged fibres. These different patterns of collagen synthesis may influence bone strength.

Bone cells

Despite their relatively small number in a large organic and inorganic tissue, bone cells dictate the structure of the skeleton. The three major cell types in bone are the osteoblasts, the osteocytes and the osteoclasts[8]. Osteoblasts, derived from fibroblastic stem cells, are responsible for the synthesis of bone matrix. They mature into osteo- cytes which lie in concentric layers within mineralized bone and serve to control local mineralization and mineral exchange between bone and plasma. Osteoclasts are multinucleate cells, derived from the monocyte–macrophage series which resorb calcified bone or cartilage. These bone cells participate in a sequential cycle of remodelling at discrete foci known as basic multicellular units[9]. At the beginning of each remodelling cycle, osteoclasts appear on a previously inactive surface and, over a period of about 2 weeks, construct a tunnel in cortical bone or a lacuna on the surface of trabecular bone. The osteoclasts are replaced by osteoblasts, which fill in the resorption cavity over a period of 3–4 months to create a new structural unit of bone. The unique aspect of remodelling is the anatomical and func- tional coupling of bone formation and resorption. In healthy young adults the two actions are tightly coupled and bone mass is maintained. Bone loss implies an uncoupling of the phases with a relative or absolute increase in resorption over formation.

THE MEASUREMENT OF BONE MASS

Early information about bone mass was obtained by *in vitro* analysis of dry, defatted skeletons, expressing results as the ash weight to volume ratio[10,11]. Although confined to autopsy specimens, these

3

TABLE 1.1   Methods of measuring bone mass

Group	Method	Site
Radiogrammetry		Metacarpal Lumbar spine Femoral neck
Absorptiometry	Single-photon	Distal forearm Mid forearm
	Dual-photon	Lumbar spine Femoral neck
	Computed tomography	Lumbar spine
	Broad-band ultrasonic attenuation	Os calcis
Overall assessment	Neutron activation analysis	Total-body calcium
	Whole-body retention of Tc-diphosphonate	Bone turnover
Histology	Dynamic bone histomorphometry	Iliac crest

studies showed that skeletal weight decreases with age above 40 years in both sexes, and in both Caucasians and Negroes. A number of non-invasive methods of bone mass measurement have subsequently been developed (Table 1.1), with varying degrees of accuracy and repeatability. These methods can be divided into four broad categories: radiogrammetry, absorptiometry, methods for the overall assessment of skeletal status and bone histology. More widespread use of these methods has led to the realization that changes in the bone mass of individuals are site-specific[12]. Cortical bone behaves differently from trabecular bone, and axial skeletal changes do not necessarily relate closely to appendicular changes. Thus, inferences about bone mass at any skeletal site from measurements made at other sites are uncertain.

Radiogrammetry

Radiogrammetric measurements have been applied to three main skeletal sites: the metacarpal, spine and proximal femur[13,14]. The major advantage of these methods is that they are simple and inexpensive.

Radiographic morphometry of the metacarpal involves measurement of the total and medullary width of the bone at its midshaft[14,15]. Measurements are made with needle-tipped calipers from hand radiographs, and may include only the second metacarpal, or a combined score from the second, third and fourth metacarpal on each side. The results are expressed as cortical width, or the ratio of cortical width to total width. Metacarpal morphometry quantifies surface-specific processes such as net endosteal resorption, but cannot reveal changes in bone tissue composition or losses due to intracortical resorption. The technique has been used to follow age-related bone loss in individuals, but is more suitable for use in population studies[16]. It correlates moderately well with the ash weight to volume ratio at the measured site, and is repeatable[16,17].

Vital assessment of biconcavity, wedging and collapse of vertebral bodies on lateral spine radiographs is subjective. Biconcavity is easily confused with artefacts due to obliquity and is of uncertain prognostic value. However, the number and degree of wedged and collapsed vertebral bodies can be assessed by a number of more objective morphometric techniques[18]. Densitometric modification of lumbar spine radiographs with the inclusion of an aluminium step wedge has also been attempted[19]. The third site at which radiographic measurements are possible is the proximal femur[13]. The trabecular bone in the femoral neck is normally arranged in a series of arches which correspond to the primary and secondary compressive and tensile stresses in the upper femur. These arches are resorbed with advancing age in an order which is determined by their functional significance. Singh suggested a six-point scale for grading the trabecular patterns, which has been shown to correlate well with the ash density of excised proximal femoral samples and to be sufficiently repeatable for use in epidemiological studies[20].

5

Absorptiometry

Photon absorptiometry was developed two decades ago as a transmission technique for measuring cortical bone in the appendicular skeleton[21,22]. A collimated beam of radiation from a radionuclide source is passed across a limb and the transmitted radiation is monitored using a scintillation detector. If soft tissue thickness around the measurement site can be made effectively constant, only one energy level of radiation is required (single-photon absorptiometry). If not, two energy levels are used (dual-photon absorptiometry).

In single-photon absorptiometry[14], the usual isotope used is iodine-125 and the limb is immersed in water. The change in beam intensity over the bone is proportional to the bone mineral content of the scanned site and may be expressed as mass per unit length or per unit area. The technique provides an accurate assessment of the amount of mineral present, with correlation coefficients of 0.98 reported with the results of ashing studies at the measured site. The repeatability of measurements is also good with coefficients of variation between 1% and 2% in normal individuals. Although any peripheral bone may be measured, the most widely adopted sites are the mid-radius (a region composed of 90% cortical bone) and the distal radius (a site containing approximately equal proportions of cortical and trabecular bone). For measurements made at the radius, there is good correlation with other cortical sites and with total body calcium assessed by neutron activation analysis. The method, however, primarily reflects changes in cortical bone and prediction of axial trabecular bone mineral content from single-photon absorptiometric measurements on the forearm is poor.

Some of the limitations of single-photon absorptiometry are overcome by making measurements at two distinct energy levels[23]. Dual-photon absorptiometry using high-activity gadolinium-153 sources has been successfully applied to measurements of the lumbar spine and femoral neck. The repeatability of spinal measurements is typically 3–5% in normal individuals and the method provides information about bone mass at key fracture sites of interest. Although the method has high accuracy, and there is a close correlation with vertebral ash density, the method also measures any other radio-opaque material within the beam, including osteophytes, aortic calcification, ligamentous calcification and previously inserted radiographic contrast media. Vertebral collapse can make interpretation difficult, so lateral spine radiographs provide a useful adjunct. The other disadvantages of the technique are its cost and the need to replace the radionuclide source every 12–18 months.

Both single- and dual-photon absorptiometry may be used to follow changes in bone mass in individuals. However, the repeatability of the measurements, although considerably better than radiogrammetric methods, still requires that measurements must be separated by considerable time intervals (say 2–3 years) to confidently detect real changes in bone mass in individuals. This problem has been reduced in recent years by the use of X-rays as the energy form, in the technique of dual energy X-ray absorption (DEXA). Measurements of the spine and proximal femur made by DEXA are considerably more repeatable than those made by DPA.

Computed tomography has been adapted to quantify bone mineral content at both appendicular and axial sites[24]. Precise location of the bone to be measured is possible, and the method has a high degree of repeatability. When applied to the lumbar spine, however, the technique measures bone and marrow resulting in poor *in vivo* validity. Recent modifications of the method, including the use of low-energy measurements and radionuclide sources, have improved this. The radiation dose is large in comparison with photon absorptiometry and the equipment is more expensive.

An alternative absorptiometric approach has recently been developed using ultrasound to assess bone mass in the os calcis[25,26]. A beam of broad-band ultrasound is propagated through the heel and its attenuation measured as a function of frequency. It has been suggested that the technique is sensitive both to the mass of trabecular bone and to its structural organization. Although preliminary results have suggested encouraging correlations between ultrasound measurements and those made by other non-invasive techniques[26], the repeatability of the method is poor, and further research is required into the precise structural characteristics of trabecular bone which are assessed.

Assessment of overall skeletal status and function

The total amount of calcium in the body can be measured *in vivo* using neutron activation analysis[23]. Following total-body irradiation of the subject by a beam of fast neutrons, small amounts of ^{48}Ca (a rare stable isotope of naturally occurring calcium) are converted to a radioactive ^{49}Ca isotope, which is measured in a total-body counter. As calcium is a constant fraction of bone mineral, ^{49}Ca can be interpreted directly as an indicator of bone mass. This costly procedure is available only in a few major research centres with irradiation facilities and whole-body counters.

The other major method for assessing overall skeletal function involves the measurement of whole-body retention of technetium-99c diphosphonate[27]. This radionuclide is thought to adsorb onto the calcium of hydroxyapatite crystals. The major factors which govern this adsorption are osteoblastic activity and skeletal vascularity. Twenty-four hours following injection, diphosphonate reaches a stable equilibrium in bone while any remaining isotope in the body has been largely cleared by the kidney. Whole-body retention provides a sensitive means of identifying increased bone turnover in a variety of metabolic bone disorders.

Bone histology

Samples of iliac crest bone may be obtained using various trocars. Conventional methods of preparing these biopsies for histological analysis entailed decalcification prior to sectioning. This procedure made distinction between mineralized and non-mineralized bone impossible, limiting the value of the method in the identification of patients with disorders of mineralization such as osteomalacia. More recently, non-decalcified sections have been made by embedding the biopsies in plastic and sectioning them with a heavy-duty microtome. The sections made in this way permit easy identification of both calcified bone and osteoid[7]. Various morphological parameters can be quantified in these biopsies, which reflect the amount and behaviour of bone in the remodelling surfaces[28]. These histomorphometric parameters also provide information about the rate of bone turnover,

8

through the quantitation of osteoclastic resorption surfaces and osteoid-covered surfaces. Finally, the dynamics of the calcification process can be studied by double-labelling the bone with tetracycline. This antibiotic binds to newly deposited bone mineral and appears as a yellow line at the calcification front when viewed under fluorescent microscopy.

Bone histomorphometry has little to offer in the diagnosis of osteoporosis, largely because of substantial within-individual variation in measurements of trabecular bone volume. It has, however, provided unique information on the heterogeneity of bone cell behaviour in osteoporosis. Furthermore, this analysis at the level of the basic structural unit of bone permits more critical choice and evaluation of therapeutic regimes in individual cases.

CHANGES IN BONE MASS WITH AGEING

Alterations in the bone mass of human beings throughout life fall into three phases: growth, consolidation and loss (Figure 1.1)[3,29].

Bone growth and consolidation

The outline of the skeleton is apparent early in foetal development and the long bones attain their future shape and proportions by about 26 weeks of gestation. Bone is formed either by the mineralization of cartilage with its subsequent replacement by bone (endochondral ossification) or directly by osteoblasts in a collagen matrix constructed by condensed layers of mesenchymal cells (intramembranous bone). The appendicular skeleton and vertebrae are formed from endochondral bone.

The newborn skeleton contains approximately 25 g of calcium[29]. If this were acquired at a constant rate throughout gestation, the demand could be met from the maternal diet. Calcium demand, however, increases towards the end of pregnancy to as much as 200 mg per day. This may be in excess of the amount absorbed by the mother, and unless dietary intake or absorption efficiency increases, the mother will lose calcium from her skeleton or the foetus will become deficient.

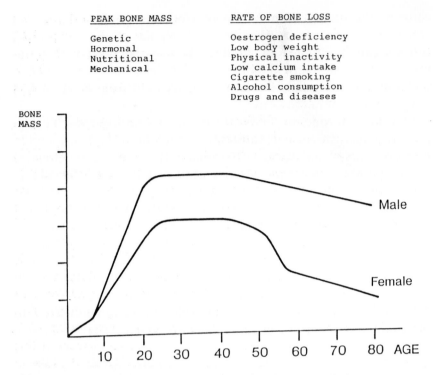

FIGURE 1.1 Diagrammatic representation of changes in bone mass with ageing and factors which influence the attainment of peak bone mass and its subsequent rate of loss

From conception to epiphyseal closure there is a progressive increase in cortical and trabecular bone mass which is accelerated during the pre-pubertal growth spurt. This growth phase produces about 90% of the peak bone mass attained during adult life. The most dramatic changes occur through linear growth of the long bones by alterations at the growth plate[30]. Studies of vertebrate limb growth have provided a model to characterize the two phases of such growth: first, the assignment of spatial orientation to the developing cells, and second, growth after these basic patterns have been laid down. During early limb development, spatial orientation appears to be influenced by adjacent ectodermal cells. Later growth seems to be autonomous and it has been suggested that this later growth is programmed during pattern formation. This later growth occurs at the cartilaginous growth plate. Here there is a stem cell population of proliferating chondrocytes arranged in parallel with the long axis of the bone. These hypertrophy and are replaced by bone. Different growth plates have characteristic rates of growth which are largely determined by the size of the proliferating zone.

Through infancy and childhood, tubular bones expand by sub-periosteal apposition and remodel by subperiosteal and endosteal resorption. These changes in bone have been studied by Garn[16,31] using metacarpal morphometry. During much of the growth period, midshaft bone gain is greater than bone resorption, resulting in a net gain of cortical bone. Photon absorptiometric measurements at the mid and distal radius have confirmed this gain in bone mass through-out childhood[32–35]. The increase is less in female than in male children, with female children having significantly lower bone mass than male children by 5 years of age, even after allowance for differences in height and weight[36]. The accretion of bone mineral during adolescence has also been defined. The spurt in bone mineral growth parallels the adolescent spurt in height. Circulating concentrations of 1,25-dihydroxyvitamin D, prolactin and sex hormones all increase at this time. In a study of 301 normal children and adolescents, Krabbe *et al.*[37] reported the timing of the adolescent growth spurt to coincide with a period of accelerated bone mineralization in both sexes. The duration of this period of rapid bone gain, however, outlasted the growth spurt. In boys the period of gain coincided with a steep increase in serum testosterone, suggesting a role for the hormone in the initiation of both linear growth and bone mineralization, and probably in the maintenance over several years of accelerated bone miner-alization. The peak increase in bone mineralization in girls was found to occur at ages 11–12 years, a time of rapidly increasing con-centrations of oestrone and oestradiol. Gonadal hormones may exert their effects on mineralization through a complex of mechanisms. First, they may have a direct inhibitory effect on bone resorption. Second, they might alter the production of 1,25-dihydroxyvitamin D and calcitonin, and third, androgens might enhance skeletal sensitivity to calcitonin.

Following the adolescent growth spurt, bone mass continues to increase for a 5–15-year period traditionally known as consolidation, during which intracortical porosity is lost and formed trabecular plates become thicker. Peak bone mass is reached during the fourth decade of life.

The formation of a bone may be affected at several stages: the condensation of primitive mesenchymal cells, the proliferation and differentiation of bone cells, the coordination of the remodelling process at cellular, tissue and organ levels[38]. Less is known of the determinants of peak bone mass. Evidence from several sources suggests a genetic potential for peak bone mass which is modified by hormonal, nutritional and mechanical factors[3]. Twin studies have shown that monozygotic twin pairs have a greater concordance for bone density than dizygotic twin pairs[39]. Correlations have been observed between bone mass values of siblings and between those of parents and children[40]. Finally, young women whose mothers have a history of vertebral fractures also have reduced bone mass. The influence of race on the incidence of osteoporotic fractures may be explained by constitutional differences in peak bone mass. Studies of Negroid populations in the USA have detected higher total bone mass than in Caucasians, whether measured by ashing studies[10] or neutron activation analysis[41]. Data from Japanese residents in Hawaii suggest lower forearm bone mineral content than in US Caucasians of similar age[42], and Polynesian women in New Zealand have been shown to have greater appendicular bone mass than Caucasians[43].

The degree to which an individual attains his or her genetic potential for peak bone mass is governed by hormonal, nutritional and mechanical factors. The major nutritional determinant of peak bone mass is probably dietary calcium intake. Approximately 400 mg of calcium are accreted into the skeleton daily throughout growth. As calcium absorption is inefficient, and there is urinary loss, calcium nutrition may become a critical factor in skeletal development. This relationship has been evaluated in a limited number of studies. Clear differences in peak bone mass were found in two Yugoslavian communities distinguished principally by a difference in calcium intake[44]. Sandler et al.[45] have more recently reported a significant relationship between cortical bone mass after menopause and milk consumption during childhood, in a large group of women. Other studies have shown that a high lifelong calcium intake is associated with greater bone mass[46,47].

The mechanical demands placed on the skeleton also influence its growth. Bone loss is a sequel of immobilization through illness[48] or space travel[49], and higher bone mass has been observed in athletic individuals[50]. In the only study to examine the interaction between calcium intake and activity as determinants of bone mass[51], independent effects of each variable were detected, but the activity effect was more marked, and related more closely to axial bone mass, while calcium intake appeared to be a preferential determinant of appendicular bone mass.

Bone loss

Skeletal growth and consolidation are followed by a transient period of stability, after which bone loss commences. This bone loss is universal. It occurs in both sexes, in all races and has been documented in prehistoric adults, be they farmers or hunters[52].

At all ages, women have lower bone mass than men, but this difference widens with advancing age. Over their lifetimes women lose about 35% of their cortical bone and 50% of their trabecular bone, while men lose about three-quarters of these amounts[3]. The differential rates of loss of cortical and trabecular bone, and the varying patterns of loss at different skeletal sites, have not been conclusively defined, largely due to a lack of longitudinal studies using sensitive methods of measuring bone mass.

A biphasic pattern of bone loss has been identified for both cortical and trabecular bone. For cortical bone[12,53], a slow phase of loss commences at around age 40 years in both sexes. The initial rate of loss is about 0.3–0.5% of peak bone mass per year, and this decreases gradually with ageing. Superimposed on this slow phase is an accelerated postmenopausal phase of cortical bone loss in women. Rates of loss during this period may be as great as 5–6% of peak per year, but they decrease exponentially to become asymptotic to the slow phase after 10 years.

Data on trabecular bone loss from the axial skeleton are less consistent[12,54–59]. For the slow phase of loss, most cross-sectional studies suggest an earlier onset of loss than for cortical bone. This phase commences in most cases at around 30–35 years, although a few studies have suggested no appreciable loss of bone until the fifth

13

decade of life. Subsequently, there is a linear or curvilinear decrease of between 0.6% and 3% of peak per year in women, and a linear decrease of 1% per year in men. Only a minority of studies have found evidence of an accelerated phase of loss in the postmenopausal decade. These findings contrast with the steep loss of bone from the lumbar spine reported after a premature menopause through oophorectomy[60].

In addition to oestrogen deficiency, many other factors may influence the rate of bone loss in individuals[61]. These include body mass, physical activity, dietary calcium intake, cigarette smoking, alcohol consumption, coexistent disease and use of certain medications.

In summary, bone mass depends on the amount of bone produced during growth and consolidation, and its subsequent rate of loss. Osteoporosis is defined as an absolute reduction in bone mass which increases susceptibility to fracture. More precise definition using photon absorptiometry or computerized tomography at axial sites has been attempted, but is difficult, as there is, at any particular age and for each sex, a wide and continuously distributed range of bone mass.

BONE MASS AND BONE STRENGTH

Bone mass is an important determinant of bone strength. Studies using cores of trabecular bone from lumbar vertebrae have shown a positive correlation between compressive strength and the ash weight to volume ratio[62]. A similar relationship between breaking stress and bone mineral content has been observed in the femoral neck[63,64]. However, variation in bone mass predicts only 40–50% of the variation in bone strength in such studies, reflecting the importance of qualitative aspects of bone structure in determining its strength. These qualitative defects may take four main forms: accumulated fatigue damage, ineffective architectural arrangement of bony elements, changes in the mechanical properties of bony materials due to ageing and osteoid accumulation[65].

Fatigue damage is a major cause of failure in structural materials. Repetitive cyclical loading of bone at strain levels below breaking strength produces such damage. However, bone differs from most inert materials in two ways. First, it is a composite of organic and inorganic material, a structural characteristic which limits propagation

14

of fatigue cracks. Second, it possesses a repair mechanism capable of removing and replacing damaged material. This protective response of bone might become impaired through defective detection of fatigue damage as a result, say, of blunted osteocyte responsiveness, or alternatively, through a defective remodelling response.

Evidence to support age-related changes in bone architecture comes from structural studies of trabecular bone using high-resolution computerized tomography. These studies show a reduction in the numbers of trabecular bars and plates with age, as well as decreased connectivity between them. These structural changes might contribute to the mechanical competence of trabecular bone.

Dickenson *et al.*[66] found a reduction in the energy-absorbing capacity of osteoporotic bone which seemed over and above the effects expected from bone loss alone. It has been suggested that this results from altered morphology of hydroxyapatite crystals and local variations in the density of osteoporotic bone.

Finally, osteomalacia – a failure of, or delay in, mineralization of newly formed bone matrix – may impair bone strength. Fractures sometimes occur in localized areas of poorly mineralized matrix, and osteomalacia has been a frequent finding in some British series of patients with hip fractures.

AGE-RELATED FRACTURES

As stated at the outset, the public health importance of osteoporosis stems from its association with age-related fractures. The most important sites at which these fractures occur are the hip, vertebrae and distal radius. However, other fractures, such as those of the proximal humerus and pelvis, may also be associated with osteoporosis. The descriptive epidemiology of these fractures is outlined below, before a discussion of the relationship between bone mass and fracture risk.

Hip fracture

More information is available on the epidemiology of hip fractures than of vertebral or distal radial fractures, largely because they enforce hospitalization. Among Caucasian women the risk of sustaining a hip fracture before the age of 90 years is estimated as one in three[67]. The

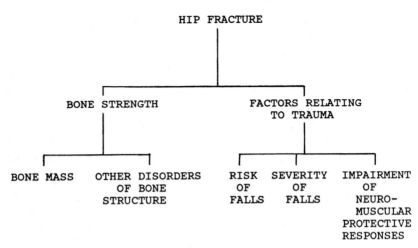

FIGURE 1.2   The pathogenesis of hip fracture in the elderly

incidence of hip fractures rises exponentially with age. Above 50 years of age there is a female to male incidence ratio of approximately 2.5 to 1. Almost 50% of hip fractures occur in individuals over the age of 80 years, and 80% occur in women. Hip fracture incidence also varies markedly with ethnic group. In those Negroid populations which have been examined, including the South African Bantu[68] and the North American black[69,70], hip fracture is infrequent and rates between men and women are equal. There are few studies of fracture rates in Oriental populations, but in Hong Kong[71] and Singapore[72] the incidence seems intermediate between that in Caucasians and in Negroids. Although the study populations have sometimes been poorly defined, and incidence estimates are therefore imprecise, it is unlikely that these ethnic variations are attributable to differences in reporting of hip fractures.

Most large studies of hip fracture in the UK have reported a winter peak in incidence[73]. Two have suggested that this peak occurs among the thinnest individuals, and is associated with falls indoors. Hypothermia, to which thin people are more susceptible, could increase the likelihood of falls by impairing neuromuscular coordination. An association between hip fracture and vitamin D deficiency during winter in the north of England provides an alternative explanation[74].

The first reliable age- and sex-specific incidence rates for hip fracture in the UK were obtained by the MRC Working Party on Fractures in the Elderly, which analysed all fractures in Dundee and Oxford during 1954–1958[75]. Since that time there has been an undoubted increase in the number of hip fractures which occur annually. Hospital admission data suggest an increase in age-specific hip fracture incidence[76], above that expected merely from the increasing number of elderly in the population. However, the use of uncorrected hospital data has been criticized on the grounds that these data are prone to error from diagnostic miscoding, readmission for late complications and inter-hospital transfer[77]. Such errors could easily have accounted for the observed increase in incidence. Recently, however, hip fractures occurring in the city of Oxford were recorded during 1 year, using the diagnostic criteria of the earlier MRC study[78]. The results showed a 35% increase in incidence over the intervening 28 years. In contrast, studies from the USA and Scandinavia suggest a plateauing in age-specific incidence rates over the last two decades[79,80].

The reason for this steep increase in hip fracture in the UK is unknown. It may reflect either a current increase in one or more environmental risk factors, or an increase in risk factors which act in early life, giving progressive increases in rates in successive generations.

Vertebral fractures

Vertebral fractures may be classified as partial (or wedge) deformities and complete (or crush) fractures. They usually occur spontaneously or following minimal trauma. Although they may cause back pain, many are asymptomatic. Vertebral fractures show a consistent predilection for two sites in the spine: the dorsal kyphus (D7–D8) and the caudal thoracic region (D12–L1)[81]. The disability and cost resulting from vertebral fractures remain unknown.

One of the few epidemiological studies carried out was a survey of 2063 ambulant female hospital outpatients and staff from South Michigan[82]. It suggested that 2.7% of women aged from 55 to 59 years had sustained one or more vertebral fractures. The prevalence rose to 20% at ages 70 to 74 years. A Danish study[83] reported that 4.5% of 70-year-old women randomly selected from the general population had crush fractures and an additional 18% had partial deformities. Estimates of crush fracture prevalence in the UK derive from female hospital outpatients in Leeds, where prevalences rise from 2.5% at age 60 years to 7.5% at age 80 years[84]. Wedge fractures are considerably more frequent with a prevalence of around 70% in women aged over 75 years.

The annual incidence of vertebral fractures in the elderly population of this country has not been directly measured. A radiological survey performed in Finland[81] using 17,557 lateral thoracic radiographs from a tuberculosis screening programme, estimated an annual incidence of thoracic spine compression fractures in women over the age of 65 years at 1.8/1000 per year, a figure comparable with a North American estimate[85] of 2.3/1000 per year among women aged 45 years and over who had densitometrically normal spinal radiographs.

Distal radial fractures

Distal radial fractures are the most common fractures in Caucasian women below 75 years of age. In the UK[86] and Sweden[87], the incidence in women has been shown to increase linearly from age 40 to 70 years. Thereafter rates stabilize. In men incidence remains constant between age 20 and 80 years. As with hip fractures, there is a winter peak in incidence. This is associated with icy weather conditions. Approximately 20% of distal radial fractures result in hospitalization, and most patients do not require intensive rehabilitation.

Hip, vertebral and distal radial fractures occur in the same individuals. Many studies have reported a greater than expected prevalence of distal radial and vertebral fractures in patients presenting with hip fractures[88]. In the Danish survey[83], the majority of patients

with vertebral fractures had also suffered one of the other two fractures.

THE RELATIONSHIP BETWEEN BONE MASS AND FRACTURE RISK

The use of non-invasive methods for measuring bone mass in patients
with fractures and non-fracture controls of similar age and sex has led
to greater understanding of the relationship between osteoporosis and
fracture risk. Reduced spinal trabecular bone mass has consistently
been found in more patients with vertebral crush fractures than in
non-fracture controls[54]. Furthermore, a threshold value can be defined
below which crush fractures occur but above which they are rarely
found. The prevalence of fractures increases the further bone mass
falls below this threshold. A reduction in spinal trabecular bone mass
therefore appears to be an important determinant of the risk of
vertebral fractures.

However, the role of osteoporosis in the occurrence of hip fracture
remains controversial. Stochastic models[89,90] can wholly explain the
variation of hip fracture incidence with age and sex on the basis of
changes in bone mass with ageing. Case–control studies, however,
have yielded inconsistent results. Fifteen studies which have examined
bone mass in patients with hip fractures and non-fracture controls
have recently been reviewed by Cummings[91]. In the six which measured
proximal femoral bone mass, values in the fracture cases were lower
than those in non-fracture controls. The difference between cases and
controls was smallest in the two studies using dual-photon absorptiometry and largest in those using grading systems of the femoral
neck trabecular pattern. The remaining studies measured cortical or
trabecular bone mass at distant sites in hip fracture cases and controls.
These failed to detect statistically significant differences in lumbar
spine bone mineral content by dual-photon absorptiometry, and two
did not detect differences in forearm bone mineral content. Such
results have fuelled the hypothesis that hip fracture risk depends more
on propensity to trauma than on bone mass. In the only case–control
study to take account of falling in its study design[92], osteoporosis was
clearly associated with hip fracture risk but other factors independent
of bone mass increased in importance with advancing age. Candidates

for these age-related factors include the previously described qualitative abnormalities in bone structure and impairment of neuromuscular mechanisms which protect the skeleton against trauma
(Figure 1.2).

Longitudinal data supporting a relationship between bone mass
and fracture have recently emerged from Hawaii[93,94]. Bone mass was
assessed by photon absorptiometry in 698 women who were followed
prospectively for up to 6 years. Low bone mass was found to be
strongly associated with the subsequent risk of developing vertebral
and non-vertebral fractures. Although the numbers of fractures on
which these risk estimates are based are currently small, the study
continues and the preliminary data have led to a resurgence of interest
in the possible use of bone mass measurements to predict fracture risk
in individuals[95,96].

CONCLUSION

Age-related fractures constitute a growing public health problem.
Current evidence suggests that osteoporosis is an important con-
tributor to the risk of these fractures. Our understanding of osteoporosis depends upon clear definition of the cellular, biochemical,
mechanical and epidemiological features of bone growth and involution. At the cellular level the skeleton must be viewed as a dynamic
organ undergoing cyclical remodelling through the actions of its con-
stituent cells. Little is known of the local regulation of this cycle and
of the mechanism whereby osteoblastic bone formation is so tightly
coupled to osteoclastic resorption. At the biochemical level an increasing awareness of the structure and properties of bone matrix is urgently
required. The biomechanical properties of bone tissue and the contribution of non-mineral bony elements to its strength also warrant
further study. Finally, the advent of non-invasive methods for measuring bone mass provides a tool with which to study bone growth and
loss in populations, enabling better definition of the factors governing
peak bone mass and its subsequent rate of loss.

Further research into all these areas is urgently required, in order
that effective preventive strategies may be designed to combat this
increasingly burdensome condition.

REFERENCES

1. Consensus Conference: osteoporosis (1984). *J. Am. Med. Assoc.*, **252**, 799–802.
2. Nordin, B. E. C., Crilly, R. G. and Smith, D. A. (1984). Osteoporosis. In Nordin, B. E. C. (ed.), *Metabolic Bone and Stone Disease* (London: Churchill Livingstone), pp. 1–70.
3. Riggs, B. L. and Melton, L. J. (1986). Involutional osteoporosis. *N. Engl. J. Med.*, **314**, 1676–86.
4. Rockoff, S. D., Sweet, E. and Bleustein, J. (1969). The relative contribution of trabecular and cortical bone to the strength of human lumbar vertebrae. *Calcif. Tiss. Res.*, **3**, 163–75.
5. Carter, D. R. and Hayes, W. C. (1976). Bone compressive strength: the influence of density and strain rate. *Science*, **194**, 1174–5.
6. Schlenker, R. A. and Von Seggen, W. W. (1976). The distribution of cortical and trabecular bone mass along the lengths of the radius and ulna and the implications for in vivo bone mass measurements. *Calcif. Tiss. Res.*, **20**, 41–52.
7. Tietelbaum, S. L. (1983). Osteoporosis and the bone biopsy. In Avioli, K. V. (ed.), *The Osteoporotic Syndrome* (New York: Grune & Stratton), pp. 115–21.
8. Russell, R. G. G., Kanis, J. A., Gowen, M., Gallagher, J. A., Beresford, J., Guilland-Cumming, D., Coulton, L. A., Preston, C. J., Brown, B. L., Sharrard, M. and Beard, D. J. (1983). Cellular control of bone formation and repair. In Dixon A. St J., Russell, R. G. G. and Stamp, T. C. B. (eds), *Osteoporosis: a Multidisciplinary Problem*. (London: Academic Press), pp. 31–42.
9. Parfitt, A. M. (1979). Quantum concept of bone remodelling and turnover: implications for the pathogenesis of osteoporosis. *Calcif. Tiss. Int.*, **28**, 1–5.
10. Trotter, M. I., Broman, G. E. and Peterson, R. R. (1960). Densities of bones of white and negro skeletons. *J. Bone Jt. Surg.*, **42A**, 50–8.
11. Arnold, J. S., Bartley, M. H., Tout, S. A. and Jenkins, D. P. (1966). Skeletal changes in aging and disease. *Clin. Orthop.*, **49**, 17–38.
12. Mazess, R. B. (1982). On aging bone loss. *Clin. Orthop.*, **165**, 239–52.
13. Singh, M., Nagrath, A. R. and Maini, P. S. (1970). Changes in trabecular pattern of the upper end of the femur as an index of osteoporosis. *J. Bone Jt. Surg.*, **52A**, 457–67.
14. Johnston, C. C. (1983). Non-invasive methods for quantitating appendicular bone mass. In Avioli, L. V. (ed.), *The Osteoporotic Syndrome* (New York: Grune & Stratton), pp. 73–84.
15. Barnett, E. and Nordin, B. E. C. (1960). The radiological diagnosis of osteoporosis. *Clin. Radiol.*, **11**, 166–74.
16. Garn, S. M. (1970). *The Earlier Gain and Later Loss of Cortical Bone* (Springfield, Illinois: Charles C. Thomas).
17. Exton-Smith, A. N., Millard, P. H., Payne, P. R. and Wheeler, E. F. (1969). Method for measuring quantity of bone. *Lancet*, **2**, 1153–4.
18. Kleerekoper, M., Parfitt, A. M. and Ellis, B. I. (1984). Measurement of vertebral fracture rates in osteoporosis. In Christiansen, C. *et al.* (eds), *Osteoporosis* 1. Proceedings of the Copenhagen International Symposium on Osteoporosis. (Copenhagen: Glostrup Hospital), pp. 103–9.
19. Nordin, B. E. C., Young, M. M., Bentley, B., Ormondroyd, P. and Sykes, J. (1968). Lumbar spine densitometry: methodology and results in relation to the menopause. *Clin. Radiol.*, **19**, 459–64.

20. Cooper, C., Barker, D. J. P. and Hall, A. J. (1986). Evaluation of the Singh index and femoral calcar width as epidemiological methods for measuring bone mass in the femoral neck. *Clin. Radiol.*, **37**, 123–5.
21. Cameron, J. R., Mazess, R. B. and Sorenson, J. A. (1968). Precision and accuracy of bone mineral determination by dual photon absorptiometry. *Invest. Radiol.*, **3**, 141–50.
22. Mazess, R. B. (1971). Estimation of bone and skeletal weight by direct photon absorptiometry. *Invest. Radiol.*, **6**, 52–60.
23. Mazess, R. B. (1983). Non-invasive methods for quantitating trabecular bone. In Avioli, L. V. (ed.), *The Osteoporotic Syndrome* (New York: Grune & Stratton), pp. 85–114.
24. Ruegsegger, P., Anliker, M. and Dambacher, M. (1981). The quantification of trabecular bone by low dose computed tomography. *J. Comput. Assist. Tomogr.*, **5**, 384–90.
25. Langton, C. M., Palmer, S. B. and Porter, S. W. (1984). The measurement of broadband ultrasonic attenuation in cancellous bone. *Eng. Med.*, **13**, 89–91.
26. Poll, V., Cooper, C. and Cawley, M. I. D. (1986). Broadband ultrasonic attenuation in the os calcis and single photon absorptiometry in the distal forearm: a comparative study. *Clin. Phys. Physiol. Meas.*, **7**, 375–9.
27. Fogelman, I. (1983). Bone scanning in osteoporosis. In Dixon A. St J., Russell, R. G. G. and Stamp, T. C. B. (eds), *Osteoporosis: a Multidisciplinary Problem* (London: Academic Press), pp. 117–20.
28. Parfitt, A. M. (1982). The contribution of bone histology to understanding the pathogenesis and improving the management of osteoporosis. *Clin. Invest. Med.*, **15**, 163–7.
29. Parfitt, A. M. (1983). Dietary risk factors for age-related bone loss and fractures. *Lancet*, **2**, 1181–4.
30. Wolpert, L. (1981). Cellular basis of skeletal growth during development. *Br. Med. Bull.*, **37**, 215–19.
31. Garn, S. M. (1981). The phenomenon of bone formation and bone loss. In De Luca, H. F., Frost, H. M., Webster, S. S. J. *et al.* (eds), *Osteoporosis: Recent Advances in Pathogenesis and Treatment* (Baltimore: University Park Press), pp. 3–16.
32. Chesney, R. W. and Shore, R. M. (1982). The non-invasive determination of bone mineral content by photon absorptiometry. *Am. J. Dis. Child.*, **136**, 578–80.
33. Landin, L. and Nilsson, B. E. (1981). Forearm bone mineral content in children. *Acta Paediatr. Scand.*, **70**, 919–23.
34. Helin, I., Landin, L. A. and Nilsson, B. E. (1985). Bone mineral content in preterm infants at age 4 to 16. *Acta Paediatr. Scand.*, **74**, 264–7.
35. Mazess, R. B. and Cameron, J. R. (1972). Growth of bone in school children: comparison of radiographic morphometry and photon absorptiometry. *Growth*, **36**, 77–92.
36. Specker, B. L., Brazerol, W., Tsang, R. C., Levin, R., Searey, J. and Steichen, J. (1987). Bone mineral content in children 1 to 6 years of age. Detectable sex differences after 4 years of age. *Am. J. Dis. Child.*, **141**, 343–4.
37. Krabbe, S., Christianses, C., Rodbro, P. and Transbol, I. (1979). Effect of puberty on rates of bone growth and mineralisation. *Arch. Dis. Child.*, **54**, 950–3.
38. Raisz, L. (1983). Regulation of bone formation 1. *N. Engl. J. Med.*, **309**, 29–35.
39. Smith., D. M., Nance, W. E., Kang, K. W., Christianses, J. C. and Johnston,

C. C. (1973). Genetic factors in determining bone mass. *J. Clin. Invest.*, **52**, 2800–8.

40. Cummings, S. R., Kelsey, J. L., Nevitt, M. C. and O'Dowd, K. J. (1985). Epidemiology of osteoporosis and osteoporotic fractures. *Epidemiol. Rev., 7*, 178–208.

41. Cohn, S. H., Abesamis, C., Yasamura, S., Aloia, J. F., Zanzi, I. and Ellis, K. J. (1977). Comparative skeletal mass and radial bone mineral content in black and white women. *Metabolism,* **26**, 171–8.

42. Yano, K., Wasnich, R. D., Vogel, J. M. and Heilbrun, L. K. (1984). Bone mineral measurements among middle-aged and elderly Japanese residents in Hawaii. *Am. J. Epidemiol.,* **119**, 751–64.

43. Reid, I. R., Mackie, M. and Ibbertson, H. K. (1986). Bone mineral content in Polynesian and white New Zealand women. *Br. Med. J., **292**,* 1547–8.

44. Matkovic, V., Kostial, K., Simonovic, I., Buzina, R., Brodarec, A. and Nordin, B. E. C. (1979). Bone status and fracture rates in rwo regions of Yugoslavia. *Am. J. Clin. Nutr.,* **32**, 540–9.

45. Sandler, R. B., Slemenda, C. W., LaPorte, R. E., Cauley, J. A., Schramm, M. M., Barresi, M. L. and Kriska, A. M. (1985). Postmenopausal bone density and milk consumption in childhood and adolescence. *Am. J. Clin. Nutr.,* **42**, 270–4.

46. Anderson, J. B. and Tylavsky, F. A. (1984). Diet and osteopenia in elderly caucasian women. In Christiansen, C. *et al.* (eds), *Osteoporosis* 1. Proceedings of the Copenhagen International Symposium on Osteoporosis (Copenhagen: Glostrup Hospital), pp. 299–304.

47. Lavel-Jeantet, A. M., Paul, G., Bergot, C., Lamarque, J. L. and Ghiania, M. N. (1984). Correlation between vertebral bone density measurement and nutritional status. In Christiansen, C. *et al.* (eds), *Osteoporosis* 1. Proceedings of the Copenhagen International Symposium on Osteoporosis (Copenhagen: Glostrup Hospital), pp. 305–10.

48. Issekutz, B., Blizzard, J. J., Birkhead, N. C. and Rodahl, K. (1966). Effect of prolonged bed rest on urinary calcium output. *J. Appl. Physiol.,* **21**, 1013–20.

49. Mack, P. B., Lachance, P. A., Vose, G. P. and Vogt, F. B. (1967). Bone demineralisation of foot and hand of Gemini-Titan IV, V and VII astronauts during orbital flight. *Am. J. Roentgenol.,* **100**, 503–11.

50. Jones, H. H., Priest, J. D., Hayes, W. C., Tichenor, C. C. and Nagel, D. A. (1977). Humeral hypertrophy in response to exercise. *J. Bone Jt. Surg.,* **59A**, 204–8.

51. Kanders, B., Dempster, D. W. and Lindsay, R. (1988). Interaction of calcium nutrition and physical activity on bone mass in young women. *J. Bone Min. Res.,* **3**, 145–9.

52. Garn, S. M., Rohmann, C. G. and Wagner, B. (1967). Bone loss as a general phenomenon in man. *Fed. Proc.,* **26**, 1729–36.

53. Smith, D. M., Khairi, M. R. A. and Johnston, C. C. (1975). The loss of bone mineral with aging and its relationship to risk of fracture. *J. Clin. Invest.,* **56**, 311–8.

54. Cann, C. E., Genant, H. K., Kolb, F. O. and Ettinger, B. (1985). Quantitative computed tomography for prediction of vertebral fracture risk. *Bone, **6**,* 1–7.

55. Krolner, B. and Pors Nielsen, S. (1982). Bone mineral content of the lumbar spine in normal and osteoporotic women: cross-sectional and longitudinal studies. *Clin. Sci.* **62**, 329–36.

56. Riggs, B. L., Wahner, H. W., Dunn, W. L., Mazess, R. B., Offord, K. P. and

Melton, L. J. (1981). Differential changes in bone mineral density of the appendicular and axial skeleton with aging: relationship to spinal osteoporosis. *J. Clin. Invest.*, **67**, 328–35.

57. Riggs, B. L., Wahner, H. W., Melton, L. J., Richelson, L. S., Judd, H. L. and Offord, K. P. (1986). Rates of bone loss in the axial and appendicular skeletons of women: evidence of substantial vertebral bone loss prior to menopause. *J. Clin. Invest.*, **77**, 1487–91.

58. Meier, D. E., Orwoll, E. S. and Jones, J. M. (1984). Marked disparity between trabecular and cortical bone loss with age in healthy men. Measurement by vertebral computed tomography and radial photon absorptiometry. *Ann. Intern. Med.*, **101**, 605–12.

59. Aloia, J. F., Vaswani, A., Ellis, K., Yuen, K. and Cohn, S. H. (1985). A model for involutional bone loss. *J. Lab. Clin. Med.*, **106**, 630–7.

60. Cann, C. E., Genant, H. K., Ettinger, B. and Gordan, G. S. (1980). Spinal mineral loss in oopherectomised women: determination by quantitative computed tomography. *J. Am. Med. Assoc.*, **244**, 2056–9.

61. Cooper, C. (1987). Individual risk factors for the development of osteoporotic fractures. *Int. Med.* (Suppl. 12), 6–8.

62. Weaver, J. K. and Chalmers, J. (1966). Cancellous bone: its strength and changes with aging and an evaluation of some methods for measuring its mineral content. *J. Bone Jt. Surg.*, **48A**, 289–308.

63. Dalen, N., Hellstrom, L. G. and Jacobson, B. (1976). Bone mineral content and mechanical strength of the femoral neck. *Acta Orthop. Scand.*, **47**, 503–8.

64. Leichter, I., Margulies, J. Y., Weinreb, A., Mizrahi, J., Robin, G. C., Conforty, B., Makin, M. and Bloch, B. (1982). The relationship between bone density, mineral content and mechanical strength in the femoral neck. *Clin. Orthop.*, **163**, 272–81.

65. Heaney, R. P. (1987) Qualitative factors in osteoporotic fracture: the state of the question. In Christiansen, C. *et al.* (eds), *Osteoporosis* 1. Proceedings of the International Symposium on Osteoporosis, Denmark, 1987 (Copenhagen: Osteopress ApS), pp. 281–7.

66. Dickenson, R. P., Hutton, W. C. and Stott, J. R. R. (1981). The mechanical properties of bone in osteoporosis. *J. Bone Jt. Surg.*, **63B**, 233–8.

67. Melton, L. J. and Riggs, B. L. (1983). Epidemiology of age-related fractures. In Avioli, L. V. (ed.), *The Osteoporotic Syndrome* (New York: Grune & Stratton), pp. 45–72.

68. Solomon, L. (1969). Osteoporosis and fracture of the femoral neck in the South African Bantu. *J. Bone Jt. Surg.*, **50B**, 2–13.

69. Gyepes, M., Mellins, H. Z. and Katz, I. (1962). The low incidence of fracture of the hip in the Negro. *J. Am. Med. Assoc.*, **181**, 1073–4.

70. Bollett, A. J., Engh, G. and Parson, W. (1965). Epidemiology of osteoporosis: sex and race incidence of hip fractures. *Arch. Intern. Med.*, **116**, 191–4.

71. Chalmers, J. and Ho, K. C. (1970). Geographic variations in senile osteoporosis. *J. Bone Jt. Surg.*, **52B**, 667–75.

72. Wong, P. C. N. (1966). Fracture epidemiology in a mixed southeastern Asian community (Singapore). *Clin. Orthop.*, **45**, 51–61.

73. Bastow, M. D., Rawlings, J. and Allison, S. P. (1983). Undernutrition, hypothermia and injury in elderly with fractured femur: an injury response to altered metabolism? *Lancet*, **1**, 143–6.

74. Aaron, J.E., Gallagher, J.C., Anderson, J.C., Stasiak, L., Longston, E.B., Nordin, B.E.C. and Nicholson, M. (1974). Frequency of osteomalacia and osteoporosis in fractures of the proximal femur. *Lancet,* **1,** 229–33.
75. Knowleden, J., Buhr, A.J. and Dunbar, O. (1964). Incidence of fractures in persons over 35 years of age: a report to the MRC working party on fractures in the elderly. *Br. J. Prev. Soc. Med.,* **18,** 130–41.
76. Gallanaugh, S.C., Martin, A. and Millard, P.H. (1976). Regional survey of femoral neck fractures. *Br. Med. J.,* **2,** 1496–7.
77. Rees, J.L. (1982). Accuracy of hospital activity analysis data in estimating the incidence of proximal femoral fracture. *Br. Med. J.,* **284,** 1856–7.
78. Boyce, W.J. and Vessey, M.P. (1985). Rising incidence of fracture of the proximal femur. *Lancet,* **1,** 150–1.
79. Melton, L.J. (1982). Fifty year trend in hip fracture incidence. *Clin. Orthop.,* **162,** 144–9.
80. Nilsson, B.E. and Obrant, K.J. (1978). Secular tendencies of the incidence of fracture of the upper end of the femur. *Acta Orthop. Scand.,* **49,** 389–91.
81. Harma, M., Heliovaava, M., Aromaa, A. and Kneckt, P. (1986). Thoracic spine compression fractures in Finland. *Clin. Orthop.,* **205,** 188–94.
82. Smith, R.W. and Rizek, J. (1966). Epidemiologic studies of osteoporosis in women of Puerto Rico and Southeastern Michigan with special reference to age, race, national origin and other related or associated findings. *Clin. Orthop.,* **45,** 31–48.
83. Jensen, G.F., Christiansen, C., Boesen, J., Hegedus, V. and Transbol, I. (1982). Epidemiology of postmenopausal spinal and long bone fractures. *Clin. Orthop.,* **166,** 75–81.
84. Nordin, B.E.C., Peacock, M., Aaron, J., Crilly, R.G., Heyburn, P.J., Horsman, A. and Marshall, D. (1980). Osteoporosis and osteomalacia. *Clin. Endocrinol. Metab.,* **9,** 177–204.
85. Iskrant, A.P. and Smith, R.W. (1969). Osteoporosis in women aged 45 years and over related to subsequent fractures. *Publ. Hlth. Rep.,* **84,** 33–8.
86. Miller, S.W.M. and Evans, J.G. (1985). Fractures of the distal forearm in Newcastle: an epidemiological study. *Age Ageing,* **14,** 155–8.
87. Alffram, P.A. and Bauer, G.C.H. (1962). Epidemiology of fractures of the forearm. *J. Bone Jt. Surg.,* **42A,** 105–14.
88. Gallagher, J.C., Melton, L.J. and Riggs, B.L. (1980). Examination of prevalence rates of possible risk factors in a population with a fracture of the proximal femur. *Clin. Orthop.,* **153,** 158–65.
89. Newton John, H.F. and Morgan, D.B. (1970). The loss of bone with age, osteoporosis and fractures. *Clin. Orthrop.,* **71,** 229–52.
90. Horsman, A., Marshall, D.H. and Peacock, M. (1985). A stochastic model of age-related bone loss and fractures. *Clin. Orthop.,* **195,** 207–15.
91. Cummings, S.R. (1985). Are patients with hip fractures more osteoporotic? A review of the evidence. *Am. J. Med.,* **78,** 487–94.
92. Cooper, C., Barker, D.J.P., Morris, J. and Briggs, R.S.J. (1987). Osteoporosis, falls and age in fracture of the proximal femur. *Br. Med. J.,* **295,** 13–15.
93. Wasnich, R.D., Ross, P.D., Heilbrun, L.K. and Vogel, J.M. (1985). Prediction of postmenopausal fracture risk with use of bone mineral measurements. *Am. J. Obstet. Gynecol.,* **153,** 745–51.
94. Ross, P.D., Wasnich, R.D. and Vogel, J.M. (1988). Detection of prefracture

spinal osteoporosis using bone mineral absorptiometry. *J. Bone Min. Res.,* **3,** 1–11.

95. Cummings, S. R. and Black, D. (1986). Should perimenopausal women be screened for osteoporosis? *Ann. Intern. Med.,* **104,** 817–23.
96. Riggs, B. L. and Wahner, H. W. (1988). Bone densitometry and clinical decision-making in osteoporosis. *Ann. Intern. Med.,* **108,** 293–5.

2

CELLULAR MECHANISMS OF BONE RESORPTION AND FORMATION

I. P. BRAIDMAN

INTRODUCTION: THE MULTICOMPARTMENTAL NATURE OF BONE

Bone is a highly complex tissue in which several different cell populations interact with one another in order to create and maintain bone structure. This is unique in the skeleton in order to withstand the mechanical forces associated with locomotion and load-bearing, and distinguishes it from other calcified tissues formed, for example, during certain pathogenic processes, e.g. calcification resulting from tissue degeneration. The different cell types signal to one another, by a variety of mechanisms, and besides intercellular relationships the matrix itself can influence bone cell function.

Bone can be divided into three major compartments: the cells which form bone (osteoblasts), those which resorb bone (osteoclasts) and the underlying bone matrix. Thus the complexity of bone structure is such that many basic aspects of its cell biology still remain unclear and are subjects for much intensive research. In this chapter contemporary views of the mechanisms by which osteoblasts and osteoclasts relate to one another, and with their underlying matrix, are discussed in relationship both to normal bone development and to pathological states.

COMPOSITION OF BONE MATRIX

Table 2.1   Composition of mammalian cortical bone[1]

	Percentage by weight		
	Fresh bone	Dry bone	Organic bone
Mineral	68.8	75.7	–
Organic	22.1	24.3	100
Water	9.1	—	–
Collagen	19.5	21.5	88–89
Non-collagenous organic	2.5	2.8	11–12
Non-collagenous components			
Chondroitin 4-sulphate	0.18	0.20	0.82
Bone sialoprotein	0.17	0.19	0.78
Insoluble CRF	0.20	0.022	0.89
α_2HS (or G_2B) glycoprotein	0.08	0.09	0.42
Albumin	0.06	0.07	0.33
Osteocalcin (or Gla protein)	0.07	0.08	0.37
Lipids	1.03	0.14	4.69
Peptides	0.12	0.13	0.53
Others	0.63	0.68	2.2–3.2

Bone has organic and mineral constituents. The organic molecules are mostly proteinaceous, as summarized on Table 2.1. Of these, collagen type 1 is most abundant, although bone sialoprotein (osteopontin), bone phosphoprotein, osteonectin (now often referred to as SPARC) and osteocalcin (bone Gla protein) are present but at much lower concentrations. Of these, osteocalcin is the only one currently thought to be bone-specific, although recent evidence[2] suggests that it may be synthesized by cultured fibroblasts. All the others are either synthesized, or their mRNA is expressed, in other tissues. Mineral is present in the form of hydroxyapatite crystals and amorphous calcium phosphate, seeded onto the collagen fibres. It is probably the folding and crimping of the collagen fibres, together with the three-dimensional relationships between the non-collagenous proteins and the mineral phase, which gives the bone its unique structure able to withstand mechanical stress and strain forces.

28

MECHANISMS OF BONE FORMATION

Is is important to understand that there are different types of bone present in the skeleton. The most familiar are the long bones, which are formed during foetal development on a cartilage anlaga. In the early stages of embryonic development the cartilage, which is originally avascular, becomes invaded by blood vessels. The chondrocytes hypertrophy, and a calcifying collar of cartilage forms, much of which is subsequently degraded and replaced by osteoblasts (bone-forming cells). This mid-region of the bone becomes the dense cortex. As bone development continues, the complexities of its structure emerge. The central bone shaft becomes traversed longitudinally by Haversian canals. These are cored out by the bone-resorbing osteoclasts, but osteoblasts follow behind them to lay down fresh bone. These canals are thought to be one of the mechanisms by which the long bones can withstand mechanical force. At either end of the long bone are the epiphyseal growth plates, where bone is less dense and of a trabecular structure. Here it is subjected to more resorption, formation and remodelling. In this region the elongation of bone occurs during the pubertal growth spurt (Figure 2.1). It contains a band of cartilage, which becomes partially invaded by blood vessels, preceding osteogenesis.

In the flat bones – which make up the skull, craniofacial areas and some regions of the vertebrae – cartilage does not participate directly in the osteogenic process, although it is sometimes present at the outer margins of the bone plates, for example in the chondrocranial regions of the calvaria during foetal development. Osteogenesis in these bones occurs by a process of 'condensation' in the mesenchymal membrane, whereby precursor osteoblasts proliferate, differentiate and lay down loosely woven bone matrix (Figure 2.2a,b). This early bone develops as a flat plate. Although it is subsequently resorbed by osteoclasts and remodelling takes place, the trabeculae characteristic of the epiphyseal growth areas of long bone do not form.

It is important to note that in mammalian development, bone is formed before marrow develops. Early stages of osteogenesis, however, occur in close proximity to microcapillary blood vessels. In the flat bones it may be seen quite clearly that the pattern of bone development parallels closely that of the small blood vessels (Figure

29

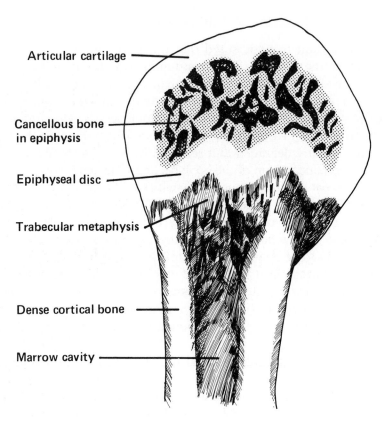

Articular cartilage

Cancellous bone
in epiphysis

Epiphyseal disc

Trabecular metaphysis

Dense cortical bone

Marrow cavity

FIGURE 2.1   Schematic diagram of a section through mammalian long bone, during a period of rapid growth.

2.3). As the bone develops the blood vessels occupy a larger area, which subsequently forms a space between the two plates of calvarial bone in the vault of the skull. This becomes the marrow space and later contains pockets of bone marrow.

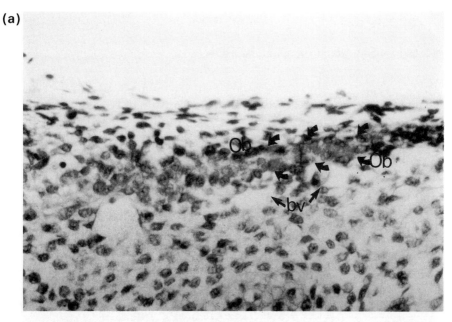

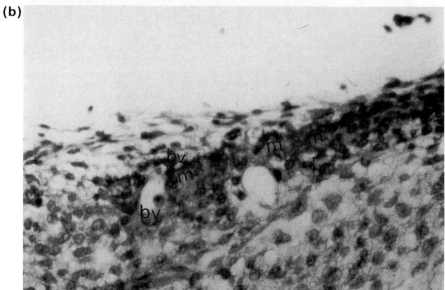

FIGURE 2.2   Initiation of intramembraneous bone formation in the fetal rat calvaria. Early 'condensation' of osteoblasts (Ob) is seen at 16–17 days gestation, shown in **(a),** with cell proliferation within mesenchymal layers (⟳). After 24 h, shown in **(b),** matrix (m) thickens as it calcifies. Note the proximity of the small capillary blood vessels (bv) (× 600).

MECHANISM OF BONE CELL ACTION

Osteoblasts

Osteoblasts form bone by laying down organic matrix (osteoid) comprising collagen type 1, osteocalcin, osteonectin, bone sialoprotein, etc. (see above). The osteoid then becomes mineralized in apposition to the direction of osteoid synthesis. The molecular steps involved in

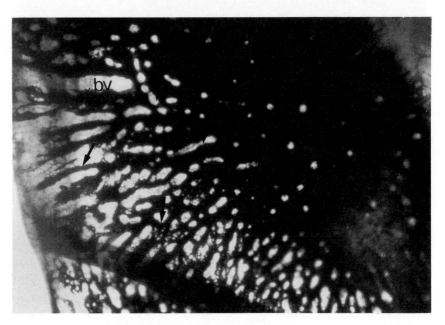

FIGURE 2.3 Mineralization patterns of flat bones. A whole fetal rat calvaria at 19 days gestation has been stained by von Kossa's method and an area of parietal bone is shown here. The calvaria is sufficiently thin and flat for microscopic inspection with transillumination, and reveals the intricate black staining pattern for the mineral (↑). The clear spaces between the whorls, loops and feather-like pattern of the bone are occupied by blood vessels (bv) (× 22).

this process are still the subject of much intensive investigation. The osteoblasts must process the mineral in some way, so that the calcium phosphate is at a sufficiently high concentration to crystallize and be precipitated onto the non-mineral bone component. Small centres of crystal formation, known as matrix vesicles[3], have been identified on

32

electron micrographs of bone and have been separated out by density gradient centrifugation from extracts of foetal bone[4]. It is thought that the vesicles form when osteoblast membrane goes through a process of 'budding off'. These vesicles have high alkaline phosphatase, pyrophosphatase and ATPase activities, together with initial high phospholipid content; thus the initiation of osteogenesis occurs extra-cellularly. It is now known, however, that osteoblast membrane contains complex ion pumping mechanisms, which may be involved in anion transport[5]. This activity may also form a considerable drain on the cells' energy supplies, and it is noteworthy that the osteoblasts are characterized by large numbers of glycogen storage granules. Bone formation and repair extend throughout the life of the individual, thereby involving constant osteoblast activity. It is important to note, however, that their activity and differentiation occurs at a rapid rate during embryonic, perinatal and pubertal periods, but in the adult their activity is more tightly controlled. The local and systemic factors which may be involved in these processes are dealt with in more detail later in this chapter.

Osteocytes

As the bone thickens, osteoblasts initially involved in bone formation can themselves become entrapped behind the advancing mineral front. These cells are then known as osteocytes and are situated within a small space or lacuna such that the mineral is never in direct contact with the cell membrane. It was thought previously that these cells were involved in bone resorption. Considerable discussion and research activity has been directed to this aspect of their function. The current consensus is that they are unlikely to be directly involved in the removal of mineral. Accurate measurements of lacuna size indicate that this is constant, and osteocyte numbers do not appear to increase in conditions of enhanced bone resorption[6]. The cells, however, have spidery processes which, after careful observation of bone histology and immunocytochemical localization of osteoblast membrane components, have been found to interconnect with one another. Their function is at present unclear, but these dendritic connections may form a communication network between the osteocytes. For example, the effect of changes in mechanical force at the bone surface could be transmitted to the inner core of the tissue by means of this osteocytic communicating network. It may also enable osteocytes to monitor conditions within the bone matrix and emit signals which could direct new bone formation or resorption. As yet there is no direct evidence to support these interesting speculations.

Cartilage cells

Chondrocytes do not form part of the mature skeleton, although they are involved in the early stages of embryonic bone formation. As discussed above, long bones are formed on a cartilage anlaga; calvariae and other craniofacial flat bones are apparently formed independently of cartilage by the process of intramembranous ossification. In the long bones, however, the cartilage cells in the region of the epiphyseal growth plate are associated with the calcification of the surrounding matrix.

It is important to note that the cartilaginous matrix secreted by these cells is quite distinct from that secreted by the osteoblasts. Chondrocytes typically secrete collagen type 2 rather than type 1, and a complex array of mucopolysaccharides which are absent in bone. Cartilage is generally under low oxygen tension, with a sparse vasculature. When calcification begins, cartilage is invaded by blood vessels, but it is uncertain whether the process of calcification is triggered by enhanced oxygenation of this tissue or factors produced by the vascular cells, or a combination of both mechanisms, resulting from the angiogenesis. Certainly recent work indicates that hyperoxic conditions prevail in the areas where calcification takes place and the cells surrounding the blood vessels produce collagen type 1, characteristic of bone[7]. It has also been thought that calcification occurs when the cartilage cells become hypertrophic and effete. It is now known that these cells are not dying, but undergoing a considerable change in their function whereby they secrete collagens, particularly collagen type 10[8], specific to cartilage undergoing the calcification process. It may be that these cells are in a different energy state to the normal 'resting' chondrocytes, perhaps due to the changes in oxygenation discussed above. The mechanism of calcification is similar to that

34

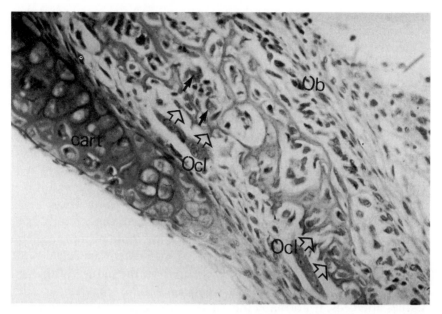

FIGURE 2.4   Osteoclasts involved in active bone remodelling. At 21 days gestation, large multinuclear osteoclasts (Ocl) are present in fetal rat calvariae, often in areas adjacent to cartilage (cart). Note the areas of bone apparently resorbed by the osteoclasts (⇧), and that smaller osteo-clasts (⬆) are also active. Osteoblasts (Ob) are laying down bone on the ectocranial surface (× 150).

described for osteoblasts, namely the formation of matrix vesicles, which is associated with an enhanced alkaline phosphatase activity[9]. One interesting hypothesis which has been put forward is that both osteoblasts and cartilage cells are derived from the same stem cell line, and at certain stages of their differentiation are interconvertible, depending on the environmental conditions (see below).

Osteoclasts

These bone-resorbing cells are classically thought of as multinuclear, similar to foreign body giant cells (Figure 2.4). There is considerable controversy at present over the exact lineage of osteoclasts and their relationship to other similar cells of the macrophage type (see below). Osteoclasts remove bone (both mineral and organic phases) from the area with which the cell is in contact, forming pits known as Howship's lacunae. The intimate contact between certain regions of the osteoclast and the bone is found by a specialized area of cell membrane known as a ruffled border, which interdigitates with the bone surface. Adjacent to these ruffled borders, which have a high concentration of lysosomes and mitochondria, are regions with few organelles, known as 'clear zones'. The function of this subcellular organization is to form a suction ring, firmly attaching the cells to the bone and it is in this area bounded by the ring that active resorption takes place. Osteoclasts have high levels of certain lysosomal enzymes, notably acid phosphatase. N-acetyl glucose aminidase, glucuronidase and succinate dehydrogenase have also been associated with osteoclast cells.

Considerable attention has been focused on the nature of the acid phosphatase enzyme present in osteoclasts. This enzyme, in other tissues and cells, is normally inhibited by sodium tartrate. It has been claimed that osteoclasts specifically contain an isoenzyme of acid phosphatase which is resistant to tartrate. Much importance has been attached to this, due to the absence of markers which will distinguish cultured osteoclasts, from similar cells, especially multinuclear giant cells, derived from macrophages. More recently, however, it has been found that the degree of tartrate resistance varies from species to species[10] and the macrophages, and cells derived from them, both *in vivo* and *in vitro*[11], also have high levels of the tartrate-resistant enzyme. Its use as a specific marker for osteoclasts must therefore be treated with caution.

The pericellular area adjacent to the resorption pit is kept at an acid pH. This has been demonstrated *in vitro* and *in vivo* by staining this region with acridine orange, a pH indicator[12], or by measuring hydrogen ion concentrations with microelectrodes. Presumably the purpose of the lowered pH is to facilitate the removal of the mineral phase of the bone. A feature of osteoclasts is the concentration of active hydrogen-ATP pumping systems in the cellular membranes and high levels of the enzyme carbonic anhydrase which generate the hydrogen ion gradient. Similar enzyme complexes are found in kidney cells.

Osteoclasts are generally thought of as multinuclear, and in fetal bone during periods of rapid remodelling there is an influx of osteoclasts onto the mineral surface. It is, however, not essential for these cells to be multinuclear, and mononuclear osteoclasts with ruffled borders and clear zones have been found to actively resorb bone.

The exact identity of the osteoclast precursors is unknown, and is the subject for much intensive investigation, which will be outlined later in the chapter. We are also unclear as to the method of osteoclast removal and disposal. *In vitro*, once these cells are separated from the bone surface, they have poor viability. This presents major difficulties for studies of osteoclasts in culture, but implies that *in vivo*, once active osteoclasts round up and are detached from the bone surface, they senesce, and this may provide an additional mechanism for controlling bone resorption.

Origin of bone cells

Until about 20 years ago there was considerable debate as to whether osteoblasts and osteoclasts were of common lineage or were derived from separate cell lines. It is now well established that osteoclasts and osteoblasts are each of distinct cell lineages; transplantation of haemopoietic cells from normal animals, to those with osteopetrosis, where osteoclasts are defective, corrects this abnormality, whereas osteoblasts are unaffected in this disorder and by this treatment[13]. In classic experiments, Kahn and Simmons[14] and Jotereau and Le Douarin[15], each showed that in embryonic quail/chick chimeras of premyeloid donors to more mature hosts, osteoclasts were of host origin. If postmyeloid donor tissue was transferred to later stage host, osteoclasts were of donor origin but osteoblast was of host origin. The results also showed that osteoblast nuclei do not contribute to osteoclasts, and that the latter were derived from haemopoietic cells. In experiments in which the circulation from the limb of one irradiated animal was transfused into the fractured limb of another shielded animal, it was shown that the osteoclast precursors were blood-borne but the osteoblasts were of a local origin[16].

Recently, Burger and colleagues[17-19] have developed an *in vitro* model system for studying putative osteoclast precursor cells, using

37

mouse embryonic metatarsal bones, from which osteoclast precursors have been removed. Their experiments indicate that mature osteoclasts can be derived from embryonic liver, spleen and yolk sac. All these tissues contain haemopoietic elements.

Osteoclasts and macrophages

Although osteoclasts are of haemopoietic cell lineage, it was thought for some time that the precursors were in fact identical to those for macrophages. The question of the relationship between macrophages and precursor osteoclasts has excited much controversy. Macrophages fuse together to form multinuclear giant cells with some characteristics similar to osteoclasts. In both cell types, maturation is enhanced by 1,25-dihydroxyvitamin D_3[20,21]. Monoclonal antibodies have been raised which were thought to be specific for osteoclasts[22,23]. Subsequently it has been found that monocytes and macrophages share common antigenic determinants[24,25], indicating a close relationship between them. We have discussed previously in this chapter some similarities in enzyme patterns, particularly with regard to acid phosphatase, in these two cell types. Calcitonin, however, is thought to have a specific effect in reducing mammalian osteoclast activity. Rodent and human osteoclasts have a large number of calcitonin receptors, although these are absent from macrophages and multinuclear giant cells[26].

Osteoclasts are also thought to be the only cells which can resorb bone. Most reports show that multinuclear giant cells, formed *in vitro* by culturing bone marrow cells, or alveolar macrophages, do not form resorption pits on the surface of bone, or the ruffled borders and clear zones characteristic of osteoclasts. Multinuclear macrophages, unlike osteoclasts, do not respond to parathyroid hormone. Although both osteoclasts and macrophages (or multinuclear cells derived from them) release radiolabelled calcium from ^{45}Ca-labelled bone, presumably by some process of resorption, the degree of similarity between osteoclasts and multinuclear giant cells is still an open question. It could still be argued that bone confers on multinuclear giant cell properties regarded as characteristically osteoclastic.

Osteoblast lineages

Although osteoblasts are known to be derived from stromal cells, the exact identity of the precursor bone-forming cells is also still uncertain. Work from the laboratories of Owen[27] and Friedenstein[28] indicates that these cells may be derived from specific clones of marrow stromal fibroblasts. In the fetus, however, bone is formed before marrow has developed. In fetal long bones a close relationship has been suggested between osteoblasts and chondrocytes[29]. In membrane bones osteogenesis is induced both before development of bone marrow and without the direct involvement of cartilage. Any hypotheses concerning the derivation of osteoblasts must also take these bones into consideration. Close observation of the development of the calvaria indicates that bone formation occurs close to the small capillary blood vessels (Figure 2.3) and it may be that there is a close relationship between the mesenchymal cells of the capillary wall (pericytes) and progenitor osteoblasts.

Cellular interactions in bone formation and remodelling

In fetal or perinatal bones, and during periods of rapid bone growth, there is active bone remodelling. In the normal adult bone the cells are generally more quiescent and under tight control. This may, of course, change under pathogenic conditions whereby bone resorption, formation, or both, are stimulated. In the long bone the trabecular region, adjacent to the epiphyseal growth plate, undergoes most remodelling. In both trabeculae and cortical bone, which contains the Haversian system, however, bone resorption is closely coupled to bone formation. Thus, when osteoclastic resorption occurs, osteoblast activity is stimulated in the resorption areas; if necessary precursor bone-forming cells differentiate and the mature cells lay down bone. Thus bone formation keeps pace with bone resorption and normal circulating calcium levels are preserved. This process is known as 'coupling' between osteoclasts and osteoblasts, and described by Frost in his concept of metabolic units of bone[30]. In the adult it is most probable that resident precursor cells are used in this process. In fetal bone, however, rapid bone formation and resorption occur, and in the early stages of bone development, osteoclasts and osteoblasts are induced *de novo*. The identity of the factors and the exact mechanism responsible for attracting in and stimulating precursor osteoblast division and mature cell activity are unknown, either in fetal or adult bone. Fetal bones, and the cells derived from them, are often used as *in vitro* systems for investigating this coupling mechanism. Results thus obtained, however, should be treated with some caution, as it is uncertain whether the mechanisms for inducing *de novo* embryonic cellular differentiation are also operating in the adult. Recent work is attempting to address this question.

Growth factors and their possible role in bone cell interaction

A variety of growth factors have recently been shown to stimulate cell division in whole bones used in organ culture systems and in osteo-blast-like cells derived from fetal or adult bones[31]. Insulin-related growth factors (IGF1 and 2) have this activity, as does skeletal growth factor. More recently this has been shown to be identical to IGF[32]. Fibroblast growth factor has also been found to stimulate mes-enchymal cell division in bones *in vitro*[33]. Some controversy exists over the action of transforming growth factors (TGFs). These were originally identified by their actions in enhancing the formation of transformed kidney cell colonies in soft agar. TGFα is thought to be similar in its activity and structure to epidermal growth factor (EGF), while TGFβ augments the effect of both TGFα and EGF in the transformed kidney cell system. Both TGFs have been associated with embryonic tissue development; TGFβ has reportedly increased cell proliferation and alkaline phosphatase activity in organ culture of bone[34] and in osteosarcoma lines[35]. Other studies[36] indicate that it has an opposite effect, so its true function in bone development is unclear. It has been suggested by Mundy *et al.*[37] that TGFβ is in fact the 'coupling factor' referred to above, and is released on osteoclastic resorption of bone to trigger osteoblast differentiation and function. He suggests that TGFβ is synthesized by osteoblasts and embedded in the bone matrix where it remains until it is activated by the acid secretions of resorbing osteoclasts and is thus able to stimulate pro-liferation of osteoblast precursors. It is important to note, however,

40

that many of these growth factors stimulate a variety of stem cell lines and types to proliferate. It is currently considered that they therefore have a major function in early embryonic growth and there is growing evidence to support this[38–40]. In the adult, many of these signals, which are part of the mechanism for rapid fetal growth, are no longer synthesized. When they are, it is usually due to pathological changes often associated with malignant disease[41]. The role of TGFβ in adult bone coupling, as expressed by Mundy et al.[37], although intriguing, should be treated with caution. Moreover, although cell proliferation is enhanced by a variety of these growth factors in osteoblast-like cell lines and in organ culture[31,33–35] there is little direct evidence of histologically recognizable bone growth and formation.

Bone morphogenic protein (BMP), or osteogenin, has been shown to induce osteogenesis. When crude extracts of bone matrix are placed under the skin of experimental animals, a small area of haemorrhage forms, around which cartilage is synthesized *de novo*. This is subsequently invaded by blood vessels, with mineralization and subsequent bone formation[31,42] Attempts to identify the active principle of BMP have been unsuccessful hitherto, and it is unknown if it consists of one or several moieties. It is important to note, however, that it is as yet the only agent capable of inducing true bone formation *de novo*.

CONTROL OF OSTEOCLASTS BY HORMONES AND OTHER FACTORS

In fetal bone there are probably many locally acting (paracrine and autocrine) factors which control osteoclast differentiation. Examination of embryonic bone development shows that there is a rapid influx of mature osteoclasts, e.g. in mouse metatarsals it occurs around 16–17 days of gestation[17] and for fetal rat calvariae it is between 20 and 21 days[43]. If either of these bones is taken before the mature osteoclasts appear, and kept in organ culture, osteoclasts mature *in vitro*, without addition of external stimuli or hormones. This indicates that there are powerful local mechanisms which promote osteoclast maturation which may, in part at least, be independent of systemic hormones. The identity of these local factors still remains uncertain;

granulocyte–macrophage colony stimulating factor (GMCSF), which has a potent effect on bone marrow, may enhance osteoclast maturation in fetal bone *in vitro*[44].

Cellular interactions in osteoclast control

Many systemic hormones and locally acting cytokines, e.g. 1,25-dihydroxyvitamin D_3, parathyroid hormone (PTH) and interleukin-1, stimulate bone resorption *in vitro*. The current view is that these molecules do not exert their effects by direct action on osteoclasts. No evidence has been found for 1,25-dihydroxyvitamin D_3 or parathyroid hormone receptors on mature osteoclasts, and it has been suggested that PTH acts on osteoclasts via osteoblasts[45]. In experiments with separated bone cells, PTH has been found to have no effect on osteoclasts if cultured alone, but does so if cultures containing osteoblasts are present[46,47]. These latter cells are known to have PTH receptors and to respond to this hormone *in vitro*. Evidence has been obtained for a soluble short-range or short-lived factor which is secreted by osteoblasts under PTH influence, which enhances osteoclast activity[46]. The exact identity of this factor still remains to be elucidated. Moreover, in fetal bone the presence of bone forming appears essential for normal osteoclast recruitment in fetal bone[18], which takes place without PTH stimulation.

Factors other than PTH – e.g. IL1[48], tumour necrosis factors α and β[49] also require the presence of osteoblasts to increase osteoclast activity. It is not known if this process is mediated by the same intercellular signals as those which appear important in the action of PTH. A further complexity in the relationship between osteoblasts and osteoclasts is the role of the underlying bone matrix. PTH has been shown to produce a retraction in osteoblast shape[50], thus exposing more bone surface. It may be that osteoclast precursors are attracted onto the mineral, and that this may also promote more maturation of these cells[51].

1,25-dihydroxyvitamin D_3 enhances bone resorption *in vitro*, and if administered to thyroparathydectomized animals, numbers of osteoclasts also increase[52]. The sterol also has effects on osteoblasts *in vitro*; it may stimulate cell proliferation and alkaline phosphatase activity[53] but can have opposite effects depending on the phenotype of cells and their culture conditions[54,55]. In any event, its true *in vivo* action on bone is often difficult to dissect out from the effects of PTH. Previously it was thought that 1,25-dihydroxyvitamin D_3 had its major action in response to hypocalcaemia, when, as a result of PTH action on the kidneys, it was synthesized and acted principally on the gut to stimulate calcium absorption, so restoring normal circulating calcium levels. Its effect on bone was also regarded as part of this system since it promoted bone resorption. More recently, however, it has been found that many cell types other than those in the intestine, bone and kidney have receptors for 1,25-dihydroxyvitamin D_3, and respond biologically to it. The sterol modifies the proliferation of precursor cells and enhances cellular differentiation and maturation[21]. For example, 1,25-dihydroxyvitamin D_3 inhibited the proliferation of the myeloid leukaemic cell line, HL60, and induced the enzymes and genes characteristic of mature macrophages[56]. Similar evidence for enhancement of osteoclast maturation by 1,25-dihydroxyvitamin D_3 has been found in some bone marrow cultures[57] and cultured fetal rat calvaria[21]. It may be that 1,25-dihydroxyvitamin D_3 enhances maturation of both bone-forming and bone-resorbing cells. Whether bone formation or bone resorption predominates as a result, may depend on the stage of bone development in the target tissue.

Calcitonin has already been referred to in this chapter as an inhibitor of osteoclastic bone resorption, and is one of the few agents which act directly on osteoclasts. It is generally thought that calcitonin operates through the adenylate cyclase system[58]. PTH was believed to act on osteoblasts by raising cyclic AMP[59]. More recently, however, calcium has been shown to be an intracellular messenger for this hormone, which is independent of adenylate cyclase[60]. Prostaglandins also increase bone resorption in organ culture, evidently by raised adenylate cyclase activity[61]. Further complexities to understanding the action of prostaglandins on bone cells have been raised by reports that prostaglandins inhibit disaggregated osteoclasts, through a mechanism which probably involves adenylate cyclase[62,63].

METHODOLOGICAL PROBLEMS IN INVESTIGATING OSTEOBLAST AND OSTEOCLAST RELATIONSHIPS

A major problem with much of the work on separated cells is that, once osteoclasts are removed from the bone surface and cultured, they are extremely fragile. Low yields of 10% live cells are currently quoted in the literature[63]. There must be some uncertainty as to whether the small proportion of cells which survive the isolation procedures are themselves viable for long periods of time in culture, or are representative of the whole osteoclast population. Methods of obtaining osteoclasts by fusion of their presumptive precursors from bone marrow have been criticized on the grounds that only multinuclear macrophages are produced by this procedure rather than true osteoclasts. Our increasing knowledge of the origin of the osteoclasts, and the concomitant availability of better and more specific markers for these cells, will help to overcome these problems.

The differences between the rapid cellular inductions occurring in fetal bone and the slower, more lightly controlled processes characterizing adult bone have been discussed previously in this chapter. We have little knowledge as to the exact nature of the hormonal and local factors which operate to control early bone induction. For example, we often use fetal bone to study the actions of PTH, but this model may be inappropriate, since its importance for fetal bone development is unclear. Of considerable importance are studies on humoral hypercalcaemia of malignancy. Patients with this condition often have a squamous cell carcinoma which secretes factor(s) which act at either the bone or the kidney level (or both), and this results in a high level of circulating calcium. A peptide related to PTH, PTH-related peptide (PTHrp) has been extracted from cell lines derived from these patients which exert these effects[64]. It has also been found to be important in fetal development by maintaining it in a state of hypercalcaemia relative to the maternal circulation[65]. It may be that PTHrp gene expression is repressed in the normal adult, but it is synthesized only in cases of neoplastic disease resulting in humoral hypercalcaemia of malignancy.

FUTURE DEVELOPMENTS IN BONE CELL RESEARCH IN RELATION TO UNDERSTANDING BONE DISEASE

Despite the problems outlined above, our understanding of the cellular interactions in bone is gradually growing. The advent of increased knowledge of the growth factors (TGFs, IGFs and CSFs) will lead to exciting prospects in our understanding of the rapid induction of bone formation and osteoclastic maturation which occur in fetal bone development. In normal adult bone these factors are probably controlled tightly, and in some cases their synthesis may even be switched off.

An important aspect of control in the adult is probably the coupling mechanism whereby osteoclasts stimulate osteoblasts by the coupling mechanism discussed above. It is important to note that, even in diseases such as Paget's disease, where there is rampant osteoclast activity in the osteolytic stage, osteoblast activity keeps pace with this. Paget's disease is probably caused by a viral infection of osteoclasts which affects precursor cells, and is transmitted to the mature multinuclear osteoclasts. The results are increased osteoclast number and activity. It is also possible that the viral infection results in a longer half-life of these cells.

In other bone disorders – for example maligant metastatic disease – the mechanism for stimulation of bone cell differentiation is equally complex. In breast cancers osteolytic metastases are common, and prostaglandins have been implicated in the mechanism of osteoclast stimulation, but more recently evidence has been presented for the stimulation of osteoclasts in this disorder by proteinaceous factors. Current thinking regarding malignant diseases is that factors important in fetal development, which are normally not synthesized in adult life, are switched on in these diseases. It may be that TGFα and β, the IGFs and CSFs may be viewed in this light, and that they may be important in understanding malignant disease of adult bone, e.g. in the formation of secondary metastatic bone lesions in breast or prostatic carcinoma.

REFERENCES

1. Vaughan, J. M. (1982). *The Physiology of Bone*, 3rd edn (Clarendon Press, Oxford), chap. 3, p. 59.
2. Bradbeer, J. N., Triffit, J., Virdi, A., Reeve, J. and Delmas, P. D. (1988). Expression of an epitope recognised by BGP/osteocalcin antisera in cultured fibroblast-like cells from human bone and skin. Presented at the Bone and Tooth Society Meeting, 23 September, Cardiff, UK.
3. Dougherty, W. J. (1978). The occurrence of amorphous mineral deposits in association with the plasma membrane of active osteoblasts in rat and mouse alveolar bone. *Metab. Bone Dis. Rel. Res.*, **1**, 119–23.
4. Bab, J., Deutsch, D., Schwartz, Z., Muhlrad, A. and Sela, J. (1983). Correlative morphometric and biochemical analysis of purified extracellular matrix vesicles from rat alveolar bone. *Calcif. Tiss. Int.*, **35**, 320–6.
5. Kellokumpu, S., Neft, L., Lopito, R. and Bacon, R (1988). The Golgi membranes of osteoblasts contain a 115 k D protein related to the anion transporter (erythrocyte band). *J. Bone Mineral Res.*, **3** (Suppl 1), 549.
6. Boyde, A. (1980). Evidence against osteocytic osteolysis. In Jee, W. S. S. and Parfitt, A. M. (eds), *Bone Histomorphometry*, (Paris: Societé Nouvelles de Publications Médicales et Dentaires), pp. 239–56.
7. Haselgrove, J. C., Golub, E. E., Chance, B., Piddington, C., Oshima, O., Tuncay, O. C. and Shapiro, I. M. (1988). Linkage between energy status of perivascular cells and mineralisation of the chick growth cartilage. *J. Bone Mineral Res.*, **3** (Suppl. 1), 460.
8. Gibson, G. J. and Flint, M. H. (1985). Type X collagen synthesis by chick sternal cartilage and its relationship to endochondrial development. *J. Cell. Biol.*, **101**, 277–84.
9. Wamer, G. P., Hubbard, H. L., Lloyd, G. C. and Wuthier, R. E. (1983). ^{32}Pi- and ^{45}Ca-metabolism by matrix vesicle-enriched microsomes prepared from chicken epiphyseal cartilage by isosmotic Percoll density gradient fractionation. *Calcif. Tiss. Int.*, **35**, 327–38.
10. Webber, D. M., Robertson, W. R., Anderson, D. C. and Braidman, I. P. (1988). A re-evaluation of tartrate resistant acid phosphatase activity in rat calvarial osteoclasts. *J. Bone Mineral Res.* (In press).
11. Oursler, M. J., Salino-Hugg, T., Wilkemeyer, M. and Osdoby, P. (1987). Soluble bone factors induce osteoclast expression *in vitro*. *J. Bone Mineral Res.*, **2** (Suppl), 258.
12. Baron, R., Neff, L., Louvard, D. and Courboy, P. J. (1985). Cell-mediated extracellular acidification and bone resorption: evidence for a low pH in resorbing lacunae and localisation of a 100 D lysosomal membrane protein at the osteoclast ruffled border. *J. Cell. Biol.*, **101**, 2210–22.
13. Loutit, J. F. and Nisbett, N. W. (1979). Resorption of bone. *Lancet*, **2**, 26–8.
14. Kahn, A. J. and Simmons, D. J. (1975). Investigation of cell lineage in bone using a chimera of chick and quail tissue. *Nature*, **258**, 325–7.
15. Joterau, F. V. and Le Douarin, N. M. (1978). The developmental relationship between osteocytes and osteoblasts, a study using quail-chick nuclear marker in endochondrial ossification. *Develop. Biol.*, **63**, 233–65.
16. Gothlin, G. and Ericsson, J. L. E. (1976). The osteoclast. *Clin. Orthop. Rel. Res.*, **120**, 201–31.

17. Burger, E. H., van der Meer, J. W. M., van de Gevel, J. S., Gribnau, J. C., Thesnigh, C. W. and van Furth, R. (1982). *In vitro* formation of osteoclasts from long term cultures of bone marrow phagocytes. *J. Exp. Med.*, **156**, 1604–14.

18. Burger, E. H., van der Meer, J. W. M and Nijweide, P. J. (1984). Osteoclast formation from mononuclear phagocytes: role of bone forming cells. *J. Cell. Biol.*, **99**, 1901–6.

19. Scheven, B. A. A., Kowilavange De Haas, E. W. M., Waassenaar, A-M. and Nijweide, P. J. (1986). Differentiation kinetics of osteoclasts in the periosteum of embryonic bones *in vivo* and *in vitro*. *Anatom. Record*, **214**, 416–23.

20. Holtrop, M. E., Cox, K. A., Clark, M. B., Holik, M. F. and Anast, C. S. (1987). 1,25-dihydroxycholecalciferol stimulates osteoclasts in rat bones in the absence of parathyroid hormone. *Endocrinology*, 108, 2293–301.

21. Braidman, I. P. and Anderson, D. C. (1985). Extra-endocrine functions of vitamin D. *Clin. Endocrinol.*, **23**, 445–60.

22. Oursler, M-J., Bell, L. V., Clevinger, B. and Osdoby, P. (1985). Identification of osteoclast-specific monoclonal antibodies. *J. Cell. Biol.,* **100**, 1592–600.

23. Nijweide, P. J., Vrijheid-Hammers, T., Mulder, R. J. P. and Blok, J. (1985). Cell surface antigens on osteoclasts and related cells in the quail studied with monoclonal antibodies. *Histochemistry*, **83**, 315–24.

24. Sminia, T. and Dijkstra, C. D. (1986). The origin of osteoclasts: an immuno-histochemical study on macrophages and osteoclasts in embryonic rat bone. *Calcif. Tiss. Int.*, **39**, 263–6.

25. Webber, D., Kinkowski, M. and Osdoby, P. (1988). Osteoclast antigen expression is dependent on both mineral and non-collagenous components of bone matrix. *J. Bone Mineral Res.*, **3** (Suppl.), 123.

26. Nicolson, G. C., Moseley, J. M., Sexton, P. and Martin, T. J. (1987). Characterization of calcitonin receptors and cyclic AMP responses in isolated osteoclasts. In Cohn, D. V., Martin, T. J. and Meunier, P. J. (eds), *Calcium Regulation and Bone Metabolism* (Amsterdam: Excerpta Medica), pp. 343–348.

27. Ashton, B. A., Allen, T. D., Howlett, C. R., Eaglesom, C. L., Halton, A. and Owen, M. (1980). Formation of bone and cartilage by marrow stromal cells in diffusion chambers. *Clin. Orthop. Rel. Res.*, **151**, 294–307.

28. Friedenstein, A. J., Chailakhyan, R. K. and Gerasimov, U. V. (1987). Bone marrow osteogenic stem cells: *in vitro* cultivation and transplantation in diffusion chambers. *Cell. Tiss. Kinet.*, **20**, 263–72.

29. Weiss A., von der Mark, K. and Silbermann, M. (1986). A tissue culture system supporting cell differentiation, extracellular mineralisation and subsequent bone formation using mouse condylar progenitor cells. *Cell Differentiation*, **19**, 103–13.

30. Frost, H. M. (1980). The ADFR concept and monitoring it. In Jee, W. S. S. and Parfitt, A. M. (eds), *Bone Histomorphometry*. (Paris: Societé Nouvelles de Publications Médicales et Dentaires), pp. 317–21.

31. Urist, M. R., DeLange, R. J. and Finerman, G. A. (1983). Bone cell differentiation and growth factors. *Science*, **220**, 680–6.

32. Strong, D. D., Beachler, A. L., Mohan, S., Weigedal, J. E., Linkart, T. A. and Baylin, K. D. J. (1988). Multiple major skeletal growth factor (SGF) in RNA transcripts expressed in human bone cells. *J. Bone Mineral Res.*, **3** (Suppl. 1), 294.

33. Canalis, E. and Raisz, L. G. (1980). Effect of fibroblast growth factor on cultured fetal rat calvaria. *Metabolism*, **29**, 108–14.

34. Centrella, M., Massagne, J. and Canalis, E. (1986). Human platelet-derived transforming growth factor B stimulates parameters of bone growth in fetal rat calvariae. *Endocrinology*, **119**, 2306–12.

35. Pfeilschrifter, J., D'Souza, S. M. and Mundy, G. (1987). Effects of transforming growth factor B on osteoblastic osteosarcoma cells. *Endocrinology*, **121**, 212–18.

36. Guenther, M. L., Cecchini, M. G., Elford, P. R. and Fleisch, H. (1988). Effects of transforming growth factor B upon bone cell populations grown in monolayer or semisolid medium. *J. Bone Mineral Res.*, **3**, 269–78.

37. Mundy, G. R., Pfeilschifter, J., Bonewald, L., Oreffo, J., Roodman, D. and Seyedin, S. (1988). Proceedings of 8th International Congress of Endocrinology, Abst 5–131, Kyoto, Japan.

38. Rotwein, P., Pollock, K. M., Watson, M. and Milbrandt, J. D. (1987). Insulin-like growth factor gene expression during rat embryonic development. *Endocrinology*, **121**, 2141–4.

39. Kimelman, D. and Kirschner, M. (1987). Synergistic induction of mesoderm by FGF and TGF-β and the identification of an mRNA coding for FGF in the early xenopus embryo. *Cell*, **51**, 869–77.

40. Weeks, D. L. and Melton, D. A. (1987). A maternal mRNA localized to the vegetal hemisphere in xenopus eggs codes for a growth factor related to TGFβ. *Cell*, **51**, 861–7.

41. Marx, J. L. (1984). What do oncogenes do? *Science*, **223**, 673–6.

42. Sampath, T. K. and Reddi, A. H. (1981). Dissociative extraction and reconstitution of extracellular matrix components involved in local bone differentiation. *Proc. Natl. Acad. Sci. USA*, **78**, 7599–603.

43. Anderson, D. C., Braidman, I. P., Lacey, E., Robertson, W. R. and Jones, C. J. P. (1984). Detailed study of the appearance and location of osteoclasts in the intact foetal rat calvaria. In Cohn, D. V., Fujita, T., Potts, J. T. and Talmage, R. V. (eds), *Endocrine Control of Bone and Calcium Metabolism* (Elsevier: Amsterdam–New York–Oxford), pp. 98–103.

44. Felix, R., Elford, P. R., Stoerckle, C., Cecchini, M., Wetterwald, A., Trechsel, U., Fleisch, H. and Stadler, B. M. (1988). Production of hemopoietic growth factors by bone tissues and bone cells in culture. *J. Bone Mineral Res.*, **3**, 27–36.

45. Rodan, G. A. and Martin, T. J. (1981). Role of osteoblasts in hormonal control of bone resorption – a hypothesis. *Calcif. Tiss. Int.*, **33**, 349–51.

46. Braidman, I. P., St John, J. G., Anderson, D. C. and Robertson, W. R. (1986). Effects of physiological concentrations of parathyroid hormone on acid phosphatase activity in cultured rat bone cells. *J. Endocrinol.*, **111**, 17–26.

47. Chambers, T. J., McSheehy, P. M. J., Thomson, B. M. and Fuller, K. (1985). The effect of calcium-regulating hormones and prostaglandins on bone resorption by osteoclasts disaggregated from neonatal rabbit bones. *Endocrinology*, **116**, 234–9.

48. Thomson, B. M., Saklatvala, J. and Chambers, T. J. (1986). Osteoblasts mediate interleukin 1 responsiveness of bone resorption by rat osteoclasts. *J. Exp. Med.*, **164**, 104–14.

49. Thomson, B. M., Mundy, G. R. and Chambers, T. J. (1987). Tumor necrosis factors (α and β) induce osteoblastic cells to stimulate osteoclast bone resorption. *J. Immunol.*, **138**, 775–9.

50. Jones, S. J. and Boyde, A. (1976). Experimental study of changes in osteoblast shape induced by calcitonin and parathyroid extract in an organ culture system. *Cell. Tiss. Res.*, **169**, 449–65.

51. Reynolds, J. J., Holick, M. F. and DeLuca, H. F. (1973). The role of vitamin D metabolites in bone resorption. *Calcif. Tiss. Res.*, **12**, 295–301.
52. Holtrop, M. E., Co, K. A., Clark, M. B., Holick, M. F. and Anact, C. S. (1981). 1,25 dihydroxycholecalciferol stimulates osteoclasts in rat bones in the absence of parathyroid hormone. *Endocrinology*, **108**, 2293–301.
53. Manolagas, S. C., Burton, D. W. and Deftos, L. J. (1981). 1,25 dihydroxyvitamin D_3 stimulates alkaline phosphatase in osteoblast-like cells. *J. Biol. Chem.*, **256**, 7115–17.
54. Spiess, Y. H., Price, P. A., Deftos, L. J. and Manolagas, S. C. (1986). Phenotypic-associated changes in the effects of 1,25 dihydroxyvitamin D_3 on alkaline phosphatase and bone GLA-protein of rat osteoblastic cells. *Endocrinology*, **118**, 1340–6.
55. Majeska, R. J. and Rodan, G. A. (1981). The effect of 1,25 dihydroxyvitamin D_3 on alkaline phosphatase in osteoblastic osteosarcoma cells. *J. Biol. Chem.*, **257**, 3362–5.
56. Reitsma, P. H., Rothberg, P. G., Astrin. S. M., Trial, J., Barsahavit Hall, A., Teitelbaum, S. L. and Kahn, A. H. (1983). Regulation of the myc gene expression in HL-60 leukaemia cells by a vitamin D metabolite. *Nature*, **306**, 492–4.
57. Takaheishi, N., Mundy, G. R., Kuehl, T. J. and Roodman, G. D. (1987). Osteoclast like cell formation in fetal and newborn long-term baboon marrow cultures. *J. Bone Mineral Res.*, **2**, 311–18.
58. Chambers, T. J. and Magnus, C. J. (1982). Calcitonin alters behaviour of isolated osteoclasts. *J. Pathol.,* **136**, 27–39.
59. Partridge, N. C., Kemp, E. E., Veroni, M. C. and Martin, T. J. (1981). Activation of adenosine-3'–5' monophosphate-dependent protein kinase in normal and malignant cells by parathyroid hormone, prostaglandin E_2 and prostacyclin. *Endocrinology*, **108**, 220–5.
60. van Leeuwen, J. P. T. M., Lowick, C. W. G. M., Bos, M. P. and Herman-Erlee, M. P. M. (1987). Calcium-dependent stimulation of ornithine decarboxylase activity in rat osteosarcoma cells by PTH. In Cohn, D. V., Martin, T. J. and Meurnier, P. J. (eds), *Calcium Regulation and Bone Metabolism*, (Amsterdam–New York–Oxford: Elsevièr), pp. 211–219.
61. Atkins, D., Greaves, M., Ibbotson, K. J. and Martin, T. J. (1979). Role of prostaglandins in bone metabolism: a review. *J. Roy. Soc. Med.*, **72**, 27–34.
62. Ali, N. N. and Chambers, T. J. (1983). The effect of prostaglandin I_2 and 6a-carba PgI_2 on the motility of isolated osteoclasts. *Prostaglandins*, **25**, 603–14.
63. Vernejoul, M-C., Horowitz, M., Demignon, J., Neff, L. and Baron, R. (1988). Bone resorption by isolated chick osteoclasts in culture is stimulated by murine spleen cell supernatant fluids (osteoclast-activating factor) and inhibited by calcitonin and prostaglandin E_2. *J. Bone Mineral Res.*, **3**, 69–80.
64. Moseley, J. M., Kubita, M., Diefenbach-Jagger, H. D., Wettenhall, R. E. M., Kemp, B. E., Sura, L. J., Rodda, C. P., Ebeling, P. R., Zajae, J. D. and Martin, T. J. (1987). Parathyroid hormone related peptide purified from a human lung cell cancer line. *Proc. Natl. Acad. Sci. USA*, **80**, 1454–8.
65. Rodda, C. J., Kubota, M., Heath, J. A., Ebeling, P. R., Moseley, J. M., Care, A. D., Caple, A. W. and Martin, T. J. (1988). Evidence for a novel parathyroid hormone-related protein in fetal lamb parathyroid glands and sheep placenta: comparisons with a similar protein implicated in humoral hypercalcemia of malignancy. *J. Endocrinol.,* **117**, 261–71.

49

3

THE PATHOGENESIS OF OSTEOPOROSIS

R. M. FRANCIS

INTRODUCTION

Contrary to the popular image of the skeleton as an inert structure supporting the rest of the body, bone is a dynamic tissue which also serves as a mineral reservoir and undergoes constant remodelling throughout life. If it were not for this remodelling, then the skeleton would be incapable of increasing in size during growth, adapting to the physical stresses placed on it, or of repairing structural damage due to fatigue failure or trauma. Bone mass changes throughout life in three major phases: growth, consolidation and involution. Up to 90% of the peak bone mass is deposited during the growth phase, which lasts until the closure of the epiphyses. There is then a phase of consolidation lasting for 10–15 years, when the bone mass increases further until the peak bone mass is achieved in the mid-30s. Involutional bone loss starts shortly after this, between the ages of 35 and 40. Both cortical and trabecular bone are lost with advancing age in women and men, though the rate of bone loss differs in cortical and trabecular bone and at different anatomical sites. The initial rate of cortical bone loss is 0.3–0.5% annually in both men and women, though this increases to 2–3% in women after the menopause, before returning to the slower rate of loss 8–10 years later. The rate of trabecular bone loss ranges from 0.6 to 2.4% per year in women, and is about 1.2% per year in men[1]. In total, women lose 35–50% of trabecular and 25–30% of cortical bone mass with age, whilst men lose 15–45% of trabecular and 5–15% of cortical bone[2–5].

Osteoporosis is characterized by a reduction in the bone mass within the skeleton, and is associated with an increased risk of fracture, often after only minimal trauma[1]. The maximum load a bone can withstand without fracture is closely related to its bone mineral content[6], so the risk of fracture is largely determined by the bone mass, though the architecture of the bone must also contribute to its mechanical properties. Newton-John and Morgan[7] suggested that there was a hypothetical bone mass value, which they called the fracture threshold, below which fractures were likely to occur. Whilst this is an attractive concept, it ignores the contribution of trauma in the pathogenesis of fractures. It seems likely that the fracture threshold is not an absolute figure, but is in part determined by the physical forces applied to the bone, as bones in young adults will fracture if subjected to sufficient trauma. Nevertheless, recent work on vertebral and femoral fractures shows evidence of a threshold bone mineral density of about $1.0\,\text{g/cm}^2$, below which fractures are likely to occur[8]. The loss of bone with advancing age leads to an increased fracture incidence in both women and men, though this is generally lower at any age in men than women[1,9]. The major fractures associated with osteoporosis are those of the forearm, vertebral body and femoral neck. About 7% of women aged 60 have sustained a fracture at one of these sites, and this increases to 25% at the age of 80[9]. In contrast, the corresponding figures for men are in the region of 3% and 8% respectively[9]. The lower prevalence of fractures in men is due to a higher peak bone mass[10], a slower rate of bone loss, and possibly greater preservation of trabecular structure during bone loss. Histological studies show that age-related bone loss in women is associated with a reduction in trabecular number without change in trabecular width, whereas trabecular width is reduced with age in men with no loss in trabecular number[2]. The bone mass at any age is determined by three variables: the peak bone mass, the age at which bone loss starts and the rate at which it progresses (Figure 3.1).

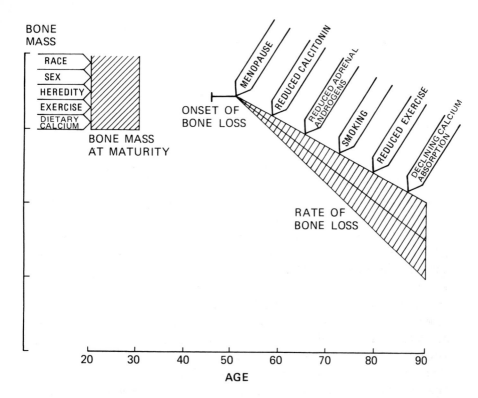

FIGURE 3.1   Schematic representation of some of the factors regulating bone mass throughout life (reproduced from Francis[4], with permission of the publishers)

PEAK BONE MASS

Peak bone mass is influenced by a number of factors, including race, sex, other genetic factors and exercise and diet during bone growth and consolidation. Negroid populations have a higher bone mass than Caucasians or Asians[11,12]. These differences are apparent early in adult life and may account in part for the observed racial variation in fracture incidence[13]. Sex is also important in determining peak bone mass, as men have bigger, denser skeletons than women[10]. Hereditary factors also influence peak bone mass, as twin studies show a greater concordance of bone mass between monozygotic than dizygotic

53

twins[14]. Exercise has a significant effect on peak bone mass, as young adults who exercise have a larger bone mass than those who exercise irregularly, and this difference is accentuated in amateur and elite athletes[15]. The bone mass is larger in the dominant arm and leg of athletes than in the non-dominant limb[15,16], emphasizing the importance of mechanical factors in the determination of bone mass. The dietary intake of calcium is another potential determinant of peak bone mass, and is particularly important as it is amenable to modification. It has been estimated that a dietary intake of about 1100 mg calcium is required daily during adolescence, because of a deposition of 300 mg in the skeleton, an obligatory loss of 300 mg calcium daily in the urine and digestive juices, and an efficiency of calcium absorption of only 55%[17]. At persistently lower calcium intakes, which are not uncommon in adolescence[18], it might be anticipated that the attainment of a maximal peak bone mass could be adversely affected. A Yugoslavian study[19] showed a higher cortical bone mass in men and women living in a region with a high mean dietary calcium intake in the range 800–1000 mg/day, than in people from an area with a low mean calcium intake (range 400–480 mg/day). The differences in bone mass were present in the fourth decade and persisted throughout life. There were also differences in the dietary intake of calories, protein, fat and phosphorus, which may have contributed to the observed differences in cortical bone mass. Nevertheless, other studies also suggest that dietary calcium intake during bone growth and consolidation influences the peak bone mass[20,21]. Hormonal factors also appear to affect peak bone mass as early menarche, pregnancy and the use of the oral contraceptive pill are associated with a higher bone mass[22].

ONSET OF BONE LOSS

Cortical bone loss starts in both men and women at about the age of 40, whilst trabecular bone loss commences between the ages of 35 and 40 in both sexes. The onset of bone loss is likely to be genetically predetermined, though how this is mediated is uncertain. It may be due to declining osteoblast function, leading to impaired new bone formation, and an inability of bone formation to match resorption[23].

This may in turn reflect the age-related decline in concentrations of systemic and local growth factors affecting bone[24].

AGE-RELATED BONE LOSS

Whilst the underlying mechanism of age-related bone loss may be a reduction in bone formation in both sexes, histological and bio-chemical studies indicate that bone resorption increases at the meno-pause, contributing further to bone loss[2,25,26]. This may account for the different changes in trabecular architecture observed with age in men and women[2]. The rate at which bone loss occurs is probably a reflection of the presence and severity of a number of factors which adversely affect bone mass. These may include the menopause, reduced circulating calcitonin, decreased adrenal androgen production, nutritional factors, smoking, reduced physical activity and declining calcium absorption (Figure 3.1). In addition, there are a number of conditions known to cause secondary osteoporosis, which aggravate age-related bone loss and may therefore accelerate the development of osteoporosis (Table 3.1).

TABLE 3.1   Causes of secondary osteoporosis

Steroid therapy and Cushing's syndrome	Amenorrhoeic athletes
	Anorexia nervosa
Myeloma	Hyperprolactinaemia
Skeletal metastases	Diabetes mellitus
Gastric surgery	Alcoholism
Anticonvulsant therapy	Immobilization
Thyrotoxicosis	Osteogenesis imperfecta
Male hypogonadism	Homocystinuria

The menopause. There is a marked reduction in the circulating concentrations of oestradiol and progesterone at the menopause, and this is associated with increased bone resorption[25-27], a more negative calcium balance[28] and a higher rate of bone loss[29,30], all of which can be reversed by oestrogen replacement[28,31-33]. Despite the clinical evidence that oestrogens inhibit bone resorption, osteoclasts appear not to possess oestrogen receptors, and physiological concentrations of oestrogen have no effect on bone resorption in tissue culture[34,35]. Alternative suggestions that the effects of oestrogens on bone resorption are mediated by changes in calcium absorption and the calcium regulating hormones[36,37] have also not been substantiated[38]. It would therefore appear that the suppression of bone resorption by oestrogens may be mediated indirectly by effects on osteoclast precursors and osteoclast recruitment, or on other non-resorptive intermediary cells such as osteoblasts or lymphocytes (see Chapter 4). In men, there are no dramatic endocrine changes in middle life corresponding to the menopause[39,40]. There may be a small reduction in plasma testosterone in later life[39,41], which may cause some bone loss, as testosterone appears to be as important for the maintenance of the skeleton in men as oestrogen is in women[42,43].

Reduced plasma calcitonin concentration. Calcitonin is a potent anti-resorptive hormone *in vitro*[44], though its physiological role in the regulation of plasma calcium and modulation of bone resorption remains uncertain. Plasma calcitonin levels are lower in women than men[45,46], and some studies show a decline in circulating concentrations with advancing age[47,48], though this is not a universal finding[45]. Although some workers have shown that oestrogen treatment increases the plasma calcitonin[36,49], this has not been substantiated by others[38,50]. It has also been suggested that osteoporotic subjects have low calcitonin levels or decreased calcitonin reserve[51], though this has not been confirmed subsequently[52,53]. Finally, it has been shown that patients with deficient calcitonin secretory reserve following subtotal thyroidectomy have no reduction in radial or lumbar spine bone mass, suggesting that the endogenous plasma calcitonin is not an important determinant of the rate of bone loss[54].

Decreased adrenal androgen producton. After the menopause the major circulating oestrogen is oestrone, produced by the conversion of the adrenal androgen androstenedione in fat[55]. Circulating androstenedione levels decline in the sixth decade of life in what has been called the adrenopause[55,56]. This may lead to a reduction in plasma oestrone[57] and further bone loss, as bone resorption in post-menopausal women is modulated by the circulating oestrone concentration[55]. The circulating levels of adrenal androgens and oestrone fall throughout adult life in men[40], though the plasma oestrone remains higher than in postmenopausal women[55], possibly protecting men against bone resorption.

Nutritional factors. A number of nutrients have been implicated in the pathogenesis of age-related bone loss, though their importance remains controversial, particularly in the case of *calcium*. There is a minimal obligatory loss of calcium in both the urine and digestive juices, and if insufficient calcium is absorbed from the diet to match this loss, calcium will be drained from the skeleton, which contains 99% of the body's calcium. The minimal obligatory loss of calcium in the urine is in the region of 50–100 mg/day, whilst the obligatory loss in the digestive juices is about 75–125 mg/day[58]. Any estimation of the dietary requirement for calcium has to take account not only of the obligatory loss of calcium, but also of the efficiency of calcium absorption, which can vary between 20% and 60% according to dietary intake[58]. The dietary requirements for calcium have been assessed by calcium balance studies, and early work suggested that the average requirement was about 500 mg/day, though 800–1000 mg/day was required to ensure that 95% of the population were in positive balance[58]. Later work suggested that a calcium intake of 1000 mg/day was necessary to prevent negative calcium balance in premenopausal women, whereas 1500 mg calcium/day was required in post-menopausal women[28]. These dietary intakes are uncommon[59-61], and it would be expected that lower intakes would lead to negative calcium balance, and loss of calcium from the skeleton. There is some evidence of a relationship between dietary calcium intake and bone mass[19-21], though this may be due to an effect on peak bone mass rather than bone loss, particularly as other studies show no relationship between calcium intake and bone mass and bone loss in postmenopausal women[62,63]. Nevertheless, calcium supplementation reduces bone resorption[64] and decreases the rate of cortical but not trabecular bone loss[65-67], suggesting that dietary calcium intake may potentially affect cortical bone loss. Some studies also suggest that the risk of femoral fracture is reduced in subjects with a higher dietary intake of calcium[19,60,61,68], though the results are a little inconsistent, and it is unclear if the apparent benefit is due to an effect on peak bone mass or the subsequent rate of bone loss. *Vitamin D* is often considered a nutrient, although the major source in humans is from cutaneous production following exposure to sunlight. The diet is normally of only secondary importance as a source of vitamin D, but becomes more significant when cutaneous production of vitamin D is restricted, as in the housebound and institutionalized elderly. In this situation, varying degrees of vitamin D deficiency may predispose to the development of osteomalacia, and aggravate age-related bone loss because of the associated malabsorption of calcium (see later). A high *fluoride* intake in drinking water may be associated with a higher bone mass[69,70], and a lower rate of vertebral and femoral fractures[69,71], though the reduction in fracture incidence is not a universal finding[70]. A high *protein* diet elevates the urinary excretion of calcium, thereby increasing the dietary requirement for calcium[72], though it is uncertain if this is a significant cause of bone loss[73]. Bone loss has been associated with low protein intakes in malnourished prisoners of war[74] and in anorexia nervosa[75], though this may be due to other factors such as low body weight, poor calcium intake and oestrogen deficiency. Nevertheless, it is likely that protein intake has little effect on bone mass, except at the extremes of protein intake[74]. Animal work suggests that a high dietary *sodium* promotes urinary calcium excretion, stimulates parathyroid hormone (PTH) secretion and increases bone resorption[76], and similar effects on urine calcium and bone resorption have been observed in postmenopausal women[77]. The significance of dietary sodium on bone loss remains unclear, however. *Body weight* may be an important determinant of bone loss, as osteoporotic subjects with femoral or vertebral fractures are lighter than expected[78,79], and bone loss in normal postmenopausal women is more rapid in women with low body weight[80]. The protective effects of high body weight on bone loss may be due to increased conversion of adrenal androgens to oestrone in fat[81], or to the mechanical effects of body weight on bone formation. Although alcoholism is a recognized cause of osteoporosis[82,83], it appears that even modest *alcohol* consumption may have an adverse effect on bone mass[84].

Smoking. Tobacco consumption is a risk factor for osteoporosis in both sexes[85,86], though the pathogenesis of bone loss in smokers is likely to be multifactorial Smoking reduces the age at menopause by several years[87], decreases plasma oestrogen levels by increasing their metabolism[88], and possibly also depresses osteoblast function[86]. Part of the deleterious effect of smoking on the skeleton may be due to the association with low body weight[85], and therefore decreased conversion of adrenal androgens to oestrone[81], as well as reduced stimulation of bone formation by mechanical forces.

Physical activity. It has long been appreciated that mechanical forces act on bone to affect trabecular architecture, but it is only recently that investigators have studied the manner in which mechanical factors regulate the production of local mediators, which modulate the cells involved in bone remodelling[89]. Physical activity is important in the maintenance of the skeletal mass, because the associated weight-bearing and muscular activity stimulates bone formation and increases bone mass[90], whilst immobilization leads to rapid bone loss[91]. It therefore appears likely that the decline in physical activity with advancing age may cause further bone loss. The importance of physical activity is underlined by several case–control studies, which show that patients with femoral fracture are habitually less physically active than control subjects[61,68,92].

Calcium absorption. The efficiency of calcium absorption from the bowel declines with age in both women and men[93], and may cause bone loss if uncompensated. Calcium absorption is regulated by vitamin D[94], and the age-related decline in calcium absorption may therefore be due to the fall in plasma 25-hydroxyvitamin D (25OHD) with age[95]. This is the major circulating metabolite of vitamin D, which is mainly derived from cutaneous production[96], with the diet acting only as a secondary source[97]. It is therefore likely that the fall in plasma 25OHD with age is largely due to reduced sunlight exposure, though inadequate dietary intake of vitamin D[98] and impaired absorption[99] and hepatic conversion of vitamin D[100] may also contribute to this. Further hydroxylation of 25OHD occurs in the kidneys to produce 1,25-dihydroxyvitamin D $(1,25(OH)_2D)$[101], the hormonally active metabolite of vitamin D which regulates calcium absorption[102]. Reduced production of $1,25(OH)_2D$ secondary to the decline in renal function with age[103,104] may therefore also contribute to the fall in calcium absorption with age. Malabsorption of calcium and low plasma 25OHD and $1,25(OH)_2D$ concentrations are therefore common in the elderly[98,105], particularly in those who are housebound or institutionalized[106,107]. Vitamin D repletion restores plasma 25OHD, $1,25(OH)_2D$ and calcium absorption into the normal range[105,108], suggesting that the decline in calcium absorption with age in the UK is due mainly to reduction of plasma 25OHD[105,108].

Nevertheless, renal impairment may also contribute to the malabsorption of calcium[105] as the elderly commonly have a glomerular filtration rate of less than 50 ml/min[109,110], and this is associated with low plasma 1,25(OH)$_2$D and malabsorption of calcium[109]. Whilst the decline in calcium absorption with age is probably due to both the reduction in plasma 25OHD and renal impairment, does vitamin D repletion affect the rate of bone loss? Nordin investigated 109 women, aged 65 to 74, who were randomly allocated to treatment with vitamin D$_2$ 15,000 units/week or placebo for 2 years. Vitamin D treatment significantly increased the plasma 25OHD into the middle of the young adult normal range, and resulted in a significant reduction in the loss of metacarpal cortical bone[111], suggesting that minimizing the age-related decline in calcium absorption by vitamin D repletion may indeed reduce the rate of bone loss. Other work shows a relationship between renal function and bone mass in the elderly[112], indicating that the decline in renal function with age may cause bone loss, possibly through decreased plasma 1,25(OH)$_2$D, reduced calcium absorption and elevation of circulating PTH[109,112,113].

ESTABLISHED OSTEOPOROSIS

Established osteoporosis is particularly associated with fractures of the forearm, vertebral body and femoral neck, and many of these will occur after only minimal trauma. Riggs has suggested that there are two distinct osteoporotic syndromes: type I or postmenopausal osteoporosis and type II or senile osteoporosis[1,114]. Type I osteoporosis presents between the ages of 51 and 75 with vertebral crush fractures and forearm fractures, and is associated with accelerated trabecular bone loss mainly due to the menopause[1]. Type II osteoporosis presents over the age of 70 with vertebral wedging and femoral fractures, and is characterized by cortical and trabecular bone loss due to age-related factors[1]. Whilst this classification may be of limited value in clinical practice, it may be useful in studies of the pathogenesis and treatment of osteoporosis, where the clinical heterogeneity of osteoporosis may otherwise lead to conflicting results. Osteoporosis may also be classified into primary or secondary osteoporosis, depending on the absence or presence of an underlying condition known to cause osteoporosis

60

(Table 3.1). This classification may be a little misleading in that it suggests that bone loss in secondary osteoporosis results from the underlying condition alone, whereas many other factors may have contributed to its development. Nevertheless such a classification may be useful clinically, as identification of a secondary cause of osteoporosis may lead to specific treatment of the underlying condition, which will prevent or even reverse the osteoporotic process. The classification of osteoporosis into primary and secondary forms may also be useful in studies of the cause and optimal treatment of osteoporosis, as these may differ considerably depending on the presence or absence of underlying conditions known to cause bone loss.

Primary osteoporosis

Of the osteoporotic patients presenting with two or more vertebral crush fractures, 65–80% of women and 45–60% of men have primary osteoporosis[1,40,115]. Women with vertebral crush fractures due to primary or idiopathic osteoporosis have reduced cortical and trabecular bone mass[9], decreased trabecular number[2] and biochemical and histological evidence of increased bone resorption compared with age-matched controls[9,26]. Both plasma oestrone and androstenedione concentrations are significantly reduced in these osteoporotic women[116], and this may account in part for their increased resorption and decreased bone mass[55]. Calcium absorption is also lower in women with crush fractures[117,118]. This may result from an intrinsic defect in the absorption mechanism[119], or from low plasma $1,25(OH)_2D$ concentrations due either to a failure of the renal 1α-hydroxylase enzyme to respond to PTH[120], or to suppression of PTH production by the calcium released by increased bone resorption [121]. Some groups have shown reduced plasma $1,25(OH)_2D$ levels in osteoporotic women[117], but this has not been confirmed by others[122]. The difference in calcium absorption between women with and without crush fractures is less marked in the elderly because of the decline in calcium absorption in normal subjects with age[93].

Men with vertebral crush fractures due to primary osteoporosis have reduced cortical and trabecular bone mass, decreased trabecular number and biochemical evidence of increased bone turnover[40] compared with age-matched controls. Although these findings are similar to those seen in women with crush fractures, there is no difference in plasma sex steroid concentrations between men with and without crush fractures[40]. Calcium absorption is, however, reduced in osteoporotic men as it is in women, and in men this appears to be due to a reduction in the plasma $1,25(OH)_2D$ concentration[40,123]. The increased bone resorption in these men with osteoporosis is slight, and probably not enough to account for the observed reduction in plasma $1,25(OH)_2D$[40].

Secondary osteoporosis

Secondary osteoporosis accounts for 20–35% of women and 40–55% of men presenting with two or more vertebral crush fractures[1,40,115]. Of the causes noted in Table 3.1, the most frequently encountered are steroid therapy, myeloma, skeletal metastases, gastric surgery, anticonvulsant therapy, thyrotoxicosis and male hypogonadism.

Steroid therapy

Although the majority of patients with Cushing's syndrome are thought to have osteoporosis[124], endogenous hypercortisolism is a relatively rare condition, not often seen in patients with established osteoporosis. In contrast, steroid therapy is the most common cause of secondary osteoporosis in patients with crush fractures[40]. The effects of corticosteroids on calcium metabolism are complex and are reviewed in Chapter 5. Steroid therapy appears to decrease calcium absorption by a direct effect on the bowel mucosa[125], resulting in some degree of secondary hyperparathyroidism and elevation of the plasma $1,25(OH)_2D$[126,127]. Exogenously administered steroids also suppress the adrenal production of androgens which consequently leads to low plasma oestrone levels[128]. As a result of these changes, the plasma levels of two bone-resorbing factors, PTH and $1,25(OH)_2D$, are elevated, whilst the plasma concentration of oestrone, a potential inhibitor of bone resorption, is reduced. In addition to these indirect actions on bone resorption, cell culture techniques suggest that steroids may also increase bone resorption by a direct effect on the osteoclast[129]. The attachment of bone-resorbing cells to bone appears to be mediated by cell surface oligosaccharides[130], and steroids may alter the expression of these cell surface sugars, thereby enhancing the attachment of the resorbing cells to bone and stimulating its degradation[129]. In addition to the stimulation of bone resorption, steroids may also suppress bone formation and collagen production[9,131]. Steroid therapy commonly causes hypercalciuria but it is unclear if this is due to the increased bone resorption or decreased tubular reabsorption of calcium[9].

Myeloma

Myeloma is characterized by extensive bone destruction, with multiple osteolytic lesions or a diffuse osteopenia, and is associated with vertebral crush fractures and pathological fractures elsewhere. The increased bone resorption is due to the production of an osteoclast activating factor by the myeloma cells[132], and recent work suggests that this is lymphotoxin[133]. A diagnosis of myeloma should be suspected in osteoporotic patients with anaemia, raised ESR, hypercalcaemia or radiological evidence of osteolytic lesions, and further investigations might include serum and urine immunoelectrophoresis and bone marrow examination. Serum and urine immunoelectrophoresis should probably be performed in all osteoporotic patients with vertebral crush fractures, as myeloma is not uncommon in these patients, even in the absence of other abnormalities on investigation. Treatment of myeloma with melphalan and steroids may improve the prognosis, particularly when given early in the course of the disease. Radiotherapy may also be helpful in patients with localized bone pain.

Skeletal metastases

The skeleton is one of the most common sites of metastases, and the bones most frequently involved are the vertebrae, femur, pelvis, ribs, sternum and humerus[134]. The tumours which most commonly metastasize to bone are carcinomas of the prostate, breast, lung, kidney, thyroid and bladder. Skeletal metastases may be either osteolytic or osteoblastic, with carcinomas of the thyroid, kidney and large bowel usually producing osteolytic metastases, whilst carcinoma of the prostate, carcinoid tumours and Hodgkin's lymphoma are associated with osteoblastic metastases[134]. Breast carcinoma may produce either osteolytic or osteoblastic metastases. The bone destruction associated with skeletal metastases may be due to the stimulation of osteoclast activity by local humoral factors released by tumour cells, or to direct resorption of bone by tumour cells[135–137]. The osteoblastic response seen with some metastases is probably due to the production of specific mitogens for osteoblasts from the metastatic tumour cells[138]. The possibility of skeletal metastases should be considered in osteoporotic patients with severe bone pain, other clinical features of malignancy, anaemia, elevated ESR, raised plasma alkaline phosphatase or hypercalcaemia. Radiology may then demonstrate osteolytic or osteoblastic lesions, and isotope bone scan may show multiple areas of increased isotope uptake. The presence of such 'hot spots' confined to the sites of crush fracture only, neither confirms nor refutes the diagnosis of metastatic disease, as any crush fracture may be associated with an osteoblastic response and therefore appear as an area of increased isotope uptake[139]. Biopsy of bone which appears radiologically abnormal, may also occasionally be useful in the diagnosis of skeletal metastases.

Gastric surgery

Although gastrectomy has long been considered a cause of osteomalacia, the precise role of gastric surgery in the pathogenesis of osteoporosis is unclear. Osteoporosis is encountered more frequently than would be expected by chance in men and women following gastric surgery[9], and in one series of men with crush fractures, 9% had a past history of gastric surgery[40]. Possible factors in the pathogenesis of bone loss after gastric surgery include decreased absorption of vitamin D, the reduced food intake which commonly follows gastric surgery, and malabsorption of calcium due to marginal vitamin D deficiency, the absence of gastric acid and intestinal hurry.

Anticonvulsant therapy

Bone densitometry indicates that bone mass in epileptic patients on anticonvulsant drugs is 70–90% of the expected value[140], and up to 8% of osteoporotic men with crush fractures are on anticonvulsant therapy, suggesting that it is a genuine risk factor for the development of osteoporosis[40]. Anticonvulsant drugs increase the hepatic microsomal metabolism of vitamin D, leading to the formation of polar biologically inactive metabolites of vitamin D, and to low plasma 25OHD levels[140]. This, together with evidence of a direct effect of certain anticonvulsant drugs on bowel mucosa, may account for the observed decrease in calcium absorption seen in patients taking anticonvulsant drugs. Anticonvulsant treatment during bone growth and consolidation may also potentially reduce the peak bone mass, and therefore lead to osteoporotic fractures in early adult life[40]. It is also important to appreciate that vertebral crush fractures may result from the trauma of convulsions rather than any underlying osteoporosis.

Thyrotoxicosis

Hyperthyroidism is associated with an increase in bone formation and resorption, though resorption usually exceeds formation such that bone is lost from the skeleton[141]. Although thyrotoxicosis is a well-known cause of osteoporosis, the diagnosis may not always be easy as elderly osteoporotic patients with thyrotoxicosis may have no other clinical features of hyperthyroidism[142]. Increased bone resorption in thyrotoxicosis leads to suppression of PTH production, low plasma $1,25(OH)_2D$ and malabsorption of calcium[141–143]. Treatment of thyrotoxicosis reverses these effects, decreasing bone resorption and increasing plasma $1,25(OH)_2D$ and calcium absorption[143]. Treatment also leads to biochemical evidence of a further increase in bone formation, which closely parallels the rise in plasma $1,25(OH)_2D$, suggesting that the initial disparity between bone formation and resorption may be due to low plasma $1,25(OH)_2D$ levels[143]. The uncoupling of bone resorption and formation during treatment of thyrotoxicosis lasts for up to a year, and might be expected to lead to an increase in bone mass and at least a partial reversal of the osteoporosis.

65

Male hypogonadism

Hypogonadism is an established cause of osteoporosis in men, and is found in 3–7% of men with vertebral crush fractures[40,43,144]. Both cortical and trabecular bone mass is reduced in hypogonadal osteoporosis[42], and histological studies show evidence of increased resorption[123,145] and decreased mineralization[42,146], which may be reversed by androgen treatment[42,123,147]. The pathogenesis of bone loss in hypogonadal men remains uncertain, though it has been suggested that it may be due to the direct effects of androgen or oestrogen deficiency[148], low plasma $1,25(OH)_2D$ concentrations[42], malabsorption of calcium[42] and reduced circulating calcitonin levels[149]. The diagnosis of hypogonadism may not always be clinically apparent in men with osteoporosis[42,123], so routine measurement of serum testosterone and gonadotrophins may be worthwhile, particularly as treatment with testosterone may partly reverse the bone loss.

Amenorrhoeic athletes

Exercise is considered to have beneficial effects on the skeleton, and athletes tend to have a higher bone mass than more sedentary individuals[15]. Nevertheless, female athletes who become amenorrhoeic have a lower than expected bone mass[150,151], and sustain stress fractures as a result[152,153]. Amenorrhoea is common in elite athletes and ballet dancers[154], occurring in up to 50% of competitive runners and ballet dancers, and is probably due to hypothalamic–pituitary dysfunction secondary to low body weight. It is therefore likely that amenorrhoeic athletes develop osteoporosis because of increased bone resorption due to low circulating oestrogen levels, in an analogous manner to that seen in young women after bilateral oophorectomy[30]. In addition to any effect on bone loss, amenorrhoeic athletes may also have a reduced peak bone mass, as many start training before the cessation of linear bone growth and experience a later than expected menarche[155]. The osteopenia observed in amenorrhoeic athletes may be partly reversible, as a reduction in training leads to weight gain, increase in circulating oestrogens, resumption of menses and improvement in bone mass[156].

Anorexia nervosa

Amenorrhoeic women with anorexia nervosa have a lower than expected bone mass[75], and develop osteoporotic fractures as a result, often in early adult life[75,157]. The osteoporosis is probably due to low plasma oestrogen levels, though dietary deficiency of calcium and protein and low body weight may contribute to the bone loss. Successful treatment of the anorexia nervosa is associated with an increase in bone mass[158], though this is likely to lead to only a partial correction of the deficit in bone mass.

Hyperprolactinaemia

Amenorrhoea is a common problem in young women[159], and is due to hyperprolactinaemia in up to 30% of cases. Women with hyperprolactinaemia and amenorrhoea have a reduction in radial and vertebral bone mass[160,161], which is most severe in those with the lowest circulating oestradiol concentrations[160], suggesting that the bone loss is due to oestrogen deficiency. Men with hyperprolactinaemic hypogonadism also have a low radial and vertebral bone mass[162,163], and may present with vertebral fractures[162]. Treatment of the hyperprolactinaemia with either surgery or bromocriptine increases bone mass in both sexes, though it appears to only partially correct the osteopenia[163,164]. It is therefore important that hyperprolactinaemia is diagnosed and treated early, to limit the loss of bone, and hopefully prevent osteoporotic fractures.

Diabetes mellitus

Osteoporosis is not generally considered to be a major complication of diabetes mellitus, though bone mass is reduced in diabetic subjects, and this is associated with an increased risk of fracture[165]. Bone loss may develop soon after the onset of diabetes[165], though its pathogenesis is unclear. Mechanisms of bone loss may include decreased bone formation due to insulin deficiency, the loss of calcium in the urine secondary to glycosuria, or increased bone resorption for other reasons.

Alcoholism

Whilst even modest alcohol consumption may have an adverse effect on bone mass[84], chronic alcoholism can lead to severe osteoporosis[82,83], and is found in 5–10% of osteoporotic men with vertebral crush fractures[40,144]. Alcoholism is associated with a decreased bone formation[83], and this may be due to a direct effect of ethanol on osteoblast function[166]. Other possible causes of bone loss in alcoholism include poor diet, malabsorption of calcium due to vitamin D deficiency, alcohol-induced loss of calcium in the urine, alcohol-related liver disease and pseudo-Cushing's syndrome. The diagnosis of alcoholism may be overlooked[167], and should particularly be considered in osteoporotic subjects who are male, have a raised MCV, abnormal liver function tests or rib fractures on chest X-ray[168].

Immobilization

As mentioned earlier, physical activity and weightbearing are essential for the maintenance of skeletal mass, and declining physical activity probably contributes to age-related bone loss. Immobilization leads to rapid bone loss of about 1% per week[90], which continues for about 6 months, when bone loss slows down and the bone mass reaches a new steady state[169]. Bone loss in immobilization is due to a stimulation of bone resorption and a decrease in bone formation[169], and this is associated with an increase in plasma calcium, hypercalciuria and possibly suppression of PTH, $1,25(OH)_2D$ and calcium absorption[170]. Immobilization leads to more rapid bone loss in weightbearing bones, suggesting that bone loss is due to local mechanical factors, rather than changes in systemic factors such as thyroxine or cortisol[170]. Therapeutic agents such as calcium and phosphate supplements, diphosphonates and thiazide diuretics have been given to prevent further bone loss in immobilization, though the results have so far been disappointing[170,171]. Where practical, remobilization should be encouraged, as this appears to increase trabecular bone mass by 0.25% per week, and may at least in part correct the osteoporosis[90].

Osteogenesis imperfecta

This is a rare and heterogeneous group of hereditary disorders, with a prevalence[172] of 1 in 20 000–50 000. The condition is probably due to abnormal collagen synthesis, composition, crosslinking and stability, and is characterized by osteoporosis, multiple fractures, skeletal deformity, blue sclerae, deafness, dental abnormalities, thin skin, cardiac abnormalities and joint laxity[173]. There are a number of classifications of the disorder based on clinical features and patterns of inheritance, but the simplest classification is into osteogenesis imperfecta congenita and osteogenesis imperfecta tarda, dependent on the age at presentation[173]. Osteogenesis imperfecta congenita is inherited as an autosomal recessive, and may lead to death *in utero* or in the neonatal period, from respiratory failure, intracranial haemorrhage or infection. Clinical findings may include a large head, soft calvarium, blue sclerae and skeletal deformity. X-rays typically show multiple fractures of different ages, deformity, osteopenia, cortical thinning and thin calvarium with multiple wormian bones. Osteogenesis imperfecta tarda is more common than osteogenesis imperfecta congenita, is inherited as an autosomal dominant, and may present with fractures in the first year of life (gravis form) or later (levis form). The condition may lead to vertebral crush fractures, loss of height and scoliosis, and fractures of the long bones may result in deformity and bowing. Blue sclerae are a common but not invariable finding and, together with osteoporosis, thin skin and joint laxity, indicates a generalized abnormality of connective tissue. Conductive-type deafness occurs in 25% of cases and is usually progressive. Dental abnormalities are uncommon, but include discoloration of the teeth, which may be small, brittle and poorly aligned (dentogenesis imperfecta). Cardiac abnormalities include dilatation of the aortic root, floppy heart valves and ruptured chordae tendinae.

Homocystinuria

This is an inborn error of methionine metabolism, most commonly due to cystathionine β synthase deficiency, which leads to accumulation of methionine and homocystine and low levels of cystathionine and cystine. It has an autosomal recessive inheritance, and an incidence of 1 in 200 000 live births[174]. Clinical features include osteoporosis, skeletal abnormality, lens dislocation, epilepsy, mental retardation, thrombotic tendency and a malar flush. The osteoporosis particularly affects the spine, and is classically associated with vertebral biconcavity, though the biconcavity tends to be posterior rather than central[175]. The long bones are also osteoporotic, with a tendency to pathological fractures which are slow to heal[174]. Other skeletal features include arachnodactyly, high arched palate, scoliosis, sternal deformity, widening of the metaphyses and enlargement of the epiphyses of the long bones, genu valgum and pes cavus[174,175]. The skeletal features of homocystinuria may be due to abnormal collagen cross-linking caused by excess homocysteine[174], and to the somatomedin-like effect of homocystine[176]. Treatment with pyridoxine may reverse the biochemical abnormalities in a proportion of patients with homocystinuria, though it is uncertain if this will improve the clinical state or prevent its progression.

REFERENCES

1. Riggs, B. L. and Melton, L. J. III. (1986). Involutional osteoporosis. *N. Engl. J. Med.*, **314**, 1676–86.
2. Aaron, J. E., Makins, N. B. and Sagreiya, K. (1987). The microanatomy of trabecular bone loss in normal aging men and women. *Clin. Orthop.*, **215**, 260–71.
3. Meunier, P., Courpron, P., Edouard, C., Barnard, J., Bringuier, J. and Vignon, G. (1973). Physiological senile involution and pathological rarefaction of bone. *Clin. Endocrinol. Metab.*, **2**, 239–56.
4. Francis, R. M. (1987). Osteoporosis in the elderly. In Hukins, D. W. L. and Nelson, M. A. (eds), *The Ageing Spine* (Manchester: Manchester University Press), pp. 18–39.
5. Horsman, A. (1976). Bone mass. In Nordin, B. E. C. (ed.), *Calcium, Phosphate and Magnesium Metabolism* (Edinburgh, London, New York: Churchill Livingstone), pp. 357–404.
6. Horsman, A. and Currey, J. D. (1983). Estimation of mechanical properties of

the distal radius from bone mineral content and cortical width. *Clin. Orthop.*, **176**, 298–304.

7. Newton-John, H. F. and Morgan, D. B. (1968). Osteoporosis: disease or senescence. *Lancet*, **1**, 232–3.

8. Riggs, B. L., Wahner, H. W., Dunn, W. L., Mazess, R. B., Offord, K. P. and Melton, L. J. III. (1981). Differential changes in bone mineral density of the appendicular and axial skeleton with aging. Relationship to spinal osteoporosis. *J. Clin. Invest.*, **67**, 328–35.

9. Nordin, B. E. C., Crilly, R. G. and Smith, D. A. (1984). Osteoporosis. In Nordin, B. E. C. (ed.), *Metabolic Bone and Stone Disease*, 2nd edn (Edinburgh, London, Melbourne, New York: Churchill Livingstone), pp. 1–70.

10. Mazess, R. B. (1982). On aging bone loss. *Clin. Orthop.*, **165**, 239–52.

11. Cohn, S. H., Abesamis, C., Yasumura, S., Aloia, J. F., Zanzi, I. and Ellis, K. J. (1977). Comparative skeletal mass and radial bone mineral content in black and white women. *Metabolism*, **26**, 171–8.

12. Reid, I. R., Mackie, M. and Ibbertson, H. K. (1986). Bone mineral content in Polynesian and white New Zealand women. *Br. Med. J.*, **292**, 1547–8.

13. Cummings, S. R., Kelsey, J. L., Nevitt, M. C. and O'Dowd, K. J. (1985). Epidemiology of osteoporosis and osteoporotic fractures. *Epidemiol. Rev.*, **7**, 178–208.

14. Smith, D. M., Nance, W. E., Kang, K. W., Christian, J. C. and Johnston, C. C. Jr. (1973). Genetic factors in determining bone mass. *J. Clin. Invest.*, **52**, 2800–8.

15. Nilson, B. E. and Westlin, N. E. (1971). Bone density in athletes. *Clin. Orthop.*, **77**, 179–82.

16. Jones, H. H., Priest, J. D., Hayes, W. C., Tichenor, C. C. and Nagel, D. A. (1977). Humeral hypertrophy in response to exercise. *J. Bone. Jt. Surg.*, **59A**, 204–8.

17. Robinson, C. J. (1987). The importance of calcium intake in preventing osteoporosis. *Int. Med.* (Suppl. 12), 28–9.

18. Hackett, A. F., Rugg-Gunn, A. J., Allinson, M., Robinson, C. J., Appleton, D. R. and Eastoe, J. E. (1984). The importance of fortification of flour with calcium and the sources of Ca in the diet of 375 English adolescents. *Br. J. Nutr.*, **51**, 193–7.

19. Matkovic, V., Kostial, K., Simonovic, I., Buzina, R., Brodarec, A. and Nordin, B. E. C. (1979). Bone status and fracture rates in two regions of Yugoslavia. *Am. J. Clin. Nutr.*, **32**, 540–9.

20. Sandler, R. B., Slemenda, C. W., LaPorte, R. E., Cauley, J. A., Schramm, M. M., Barresi, M. L. and Kriska, A. M. (1985). Postmenopausal bone density and milk consumption in childhood and adolescence. *Am. J. Clin. Nutr.*, **42**, 270–4.

21. Anderson, J. J. B. and Tylavsky, F. A. (1984). Diet and osteopenia in elderly caucasian women. In Christiansen, C., Arnaud, C. D., Nordin, B. E. C., Parfitt, A. M., Peck, W. A. and Riggs, B. L. (eds), *Osteoporosis* (Copenhagen: Glostrup Hospital), pp. 299–304.

22. Goldsmith, N. F. and Johnston, J. O. (1975). Bone mineral: effects of oral contraceptives, pregnancy and lactation. *J. Bone Jt. Surg.*, **57A**, 657–68.

23. Lips, P., Courpron, P. and Meunier, P. J. (1978). Mean wall thickness of trabecular bone packets in human iliac crest: changes with age. *Calcif. Tissue Res.*, **26**, 13–17.

24. Rudman, D., Kutner, M. H., Rogers, C. M., Lubin, M. F., Fleming, G. A. and Bain, R. P. (1981). Impaired growth hormone secretion in the adult population: relation to age and adiposity. *J. Clin. Invest.,* **67,** 1361–9.

25. Hodgkinson, A. and Thompson, T. (1982). Measurement of the fasting urine hydroxyproline: creatinine ratio in normal adults and its variation with age and sex. *J. Clin. Pathol.,* **35,** 807–11.

26. Nordin, B. E. C., Aaron, J., Speed, R. and Crilly, R. G. (1981). Bone formation and resorption as the determinants of trabecular bone volume in postmenopausal osteoporosis. *Lancet,* **2,** 277–9.

27. Nordin, B. E. C., Peacock, M., Aaron, J. E., Crilly, R. G., Heyburn, P. J., Horsman, A. and Marshall, D. H. (1980). Osteoporosis and osteomalacia. *Clin. Endocrinol. Metab.,* **9,** 177–205.

28. Heaney, R. P., Recker, R. R. and Saville, P. D. (1978). Menopausal changes in calcium balance performance. *J. Lab. Clin. Med.,* **92,** 953–63.

29. Meema, H. E. (1966). Menopausal and aging changes in muscle mass and bone mineral content. *J. Bone Jt. Surg.,* **48A,** 1138–44.

30. Aitken, J. M., Hart, D. M., Anderson, J. B., Lindsay, R., Smith, D. A. and Speirs, C. F. (1973). Osteoporosis after oophorectomy for non-malignant disease in premenopausal women. *Br. Med. J.,* **2,** 325–8.

31. Lafferty, F. W., Spencer, G. E. Jr and Pearson, O. H. (1964). Effects of androgens, estrogens and high calcium intakes on bone formation and resorption in osteoporosis. *Am. J. Med.,* **36,** 514–28.

32. Lindsay, R., Hart, D. M., Aitken, J. M., MacDonald, E. B., Anderson, J. B. and Clarke, A. C. (1976). Long-term prevention of postmenopausal osteoporosis by oestrogen. *Lancet,* **1,** 1038–40.

33. Horsman, A., Jones, M., Francis, R. and Nordin, C. (1983). The effect of estrogen dose on postmenopausal bone loss. *N. Engl. J. Med.,* **309,** 1405–7.

34. Caputo, C. B., Meadows, D. and Raisz, L. G. (1976). Failure of estrogens and androgens to inhibit bone resorption in tissue culture. *Endocrinology,* **98,** 1065–8.

35. Francis, R. M., Peacock, M., Taylor, G. A., Kahn, A. J. and Teitelbaum, S. L. (1985). How do oestrogens modulate bone resorption? In Norman, A. W., Schaefer, K., Grigoleit, H.-G. and Herrath, D.v. (eds), *Vitamin D: chemical, biochemical and clinical update* (Berlin, New York: Walter de Gruyter), pp. 479–80.

36. Stevenson, J. C., Abeyasekera, G., Hillyard, C. J., Phang, K. G., MacIntyre, I., Campbell, S., Townsend, P. T., Young, O. and Whitehead, M. I. (1981). Calcitonin and the calcium-regulating hormones in postmenopausal women: effect of oestrogens. *Lancet,* **1,** 693–5.

37. Gallagher, J. C., Riggs, B. L. and DeLuca, H. F. (1980). Effect of estrogen on calcium absorption and serum vitamin D metabolites in postmenopausal osteoporosis. *J. Clin. Endocrinol Metab.,* **51,** 1359–64.

38. Selby, P. L., Peacock, M., Barkworth, S. A., Brown, W. B. and Taylor, G. A. (1985). Early effects of ethinyloestradiol and norethisterone treatment on bone resorption and calcium regulating hormones. *Clin. Sci.,* **69,** 265–71.

39. Stearns, E. L., MacDonnell, J. A., Kaufman, B. J., Padua, R., Lucman, T. S., Winter, J. S. D. and Faiman, C. (1974). Declining testicular function with age. Hormonal and clinical correlates. *Am. J. Med.,* **57,** 761–6.

40. Francis, R. M., Peacock, M., Marshall, D. H., Horsman, A. and Aaron, J. E.

(1989). Spinal osteoporosis in men. *Bone and Mineral,* **5,** 347–57.

41. Baker, H. W. G., Burger, H. G., De Kretser, D. M., Hudson, B., O'Connor, S., Wang, C., Mirovics, A., Court, J., Dunlop, M. and Rennie, G. C. (1976). Changes in the pituitary–testicular system with age. *Clin. Endocrinol.,* **5,** 349–72.

42. Francis, R. M., Peacock, M., Aaron, J. E., Selby, P. L., Taylor, G. A., Thompson, J., Marshall, D. H. and Horsman, A. (1986). Osteoporosis in hypogonadal men: role of decreased plasma 1,25-dihydroxyvitamin D, calcium malabsorption, and low bone formation. *Bone,* **7,** 261–8.

43. Seeman, E., Melton, L. J. III, O'Fallon, W. M. and Riggs, B. L. (1983). Risk factors for spinal osteoporosis in men. *Am. J. Med.,* **75,** 977–83.

44. Chambers, T. J., McSheehy, P. M. J., Thomson, B. M. and Fuller, K. (1985). The effect of calcium-regulating hormones and prostaglandins on bone resorption by osteoclasts disaggregated from neonatal rabbit bones. *Endocrinology,* **116,** 234–9.

45. Body, J.-J. and Heath, H. III (1983). Estimates of circulating monomeric calcitonin: Physiological studies in normal and thyroidectomized man. *J. Clin. Endocrinol. Metab.,* **57,** 897–903.

46. Stevenson, J. C. (1982). Regulation of calcitonin and parathyroid hormone secretion by oestrogens. *Maturitas,* **4,** 1–7.

47. Deftos, L. J., Weisman, M. H., Williams, G. W., Karpf, D. B., Frumar, A. M., Davidson, B. J., Parthemore, J. G. and Judd, H. L. (1980). Influence of age and sex on plasma calcitonin in human beings. *N. Engl. J. Med.,* **302,** 1351–3.

48. Shamonki, I. M., Frumar, A. M., Tataryn, I. V., Meldrum, D. R., Davidson, B. H., Parthemore, J. G., Judd, H. L. and Deftos, L. J. (1980). Age-related changes of calcitonin secretion in females. *J. Clin. Endocrinol. Metab.,* **50,** 437–9.

49. Morimoto, S., Tsuji, M., Okada, Y., Onishi, T. and Kumahara, Y. (1980). The effect of oestrogens on human calcitonin secretion after calcium infusion in elderly female subjects. *Clin. Endocrinol.,* **13,** 135–43.

50. Leggate, J., Farish, E., Fletcher, C. D., McIntosh, W., Hart, D. M. and Somerville, J. M. (1984). Calcitonin and postmenopausal osteoporosis. *Clin. Endocrinol.,* **20,** 85–92.

51. Taggart, H. M., Chesnut, C. H. III., Ivey, J. L., Baylink, D. J., Sisom, K., Huber, M. B. and Roos, B. A. (1982). Deficient calcitonin response to calcium stimulation in postmenopausal osteoporosis? *Lancet,* **1,** 475–8.

52. Tiegs, R. D., Body, J. J., Wahner, H. W., Barta, J., Riggs, B. L. and Heath, H. III (1985). Calcitonin secretion in postmenopausal osteoporosis. *N. Engl. J. Med.,* **312,** 1097–1100.

53. Beringer, T. R. O., Ardill, J. and Taggart, H. M. (1986). Absence of evidence for a role of calcitonin in the etiology of femoral neck fracture. *Calcif. Tissue Int.,* **39,** 300–3.

54. Hurley, D. L., Tiegs, R. D., Wahner, H. W. and Heath, H. III (1987). Axial and appendicular bone mineral density in patients with long-term deficiency or excess calcitonin. *N. Engl. J. Med.,* **317,** 537–41.

55. Crilly, R. G., Francis, R. M. and Nordin, B. E. C. (1981). Steroid hormones, ageing and bone. *Clin. Endocrinol. Metab.,* **10,** 115–39.

56. Crilly, R. G., Marshall, D. H. and Nordin, B. E. C. (1979). Effect of age on

plasma androstenedione concentration in oophorectomized women. *Clin. Endocrinol.,* **10,** 199–201.

57. Nordin, B. E. C., Crilly, R. G., Marshall, D. H. and Barkworth, S. A. (1981). Oestrogens, the menopause and the adrenopause. *J. Endocrinol.,* **89,** 131P–143P.

58. Nordin, B. E. C., Horsman, A., Marshall, D. H., Simpson, M. and Waterhouse, G. M. (1979). Calcium requirement and calcium therapy. *Clin. Orthop.,* **140,** 216–39.

59. Heaney, R. P., Gallagher, J. C., Johnston, C. C., Neer, R., Parfitt, A. M. and Whedon, G. D. (1982). Calcium nutrition and bone health in the elderly. *Am. J. Clin. Nutr.,* **36,** 986–1013.

60. Holbrook, T. L., Barrett-Connor, E. and Wingard, D. L. (1988). Dietary calcium and risk of hip fracture: 14-year prospective population study. *Lancet,* **2,** 1046–9.

61. Cooper, C., Barker, D. J. P. and Wickham, C. (1988). Physical activity, muscle strength, and calcium intake in fracture of the proximal femur in Britain. *Br. Med. J.,* **297,** 1443–6.

62. Riggs, B. L., Wahner, H. W., Melton, L. J. III, Richelson, L. S., Judd, H. L. and O'Fallon, W. M. (1987). Dietary calcium intake and rates of bone loss in women. *J. Clin. Invest.,* **80,** 979–82.

63. Stevenson, J. C., Whitehead, M. I., Padwick, M., Endacott, J. A., Sutton, C., Banks, L. M., Freemantle, C., Spinks, T. J. and Hesp, R. (1988). Dietary intake of calcium and postmenopausal bone loss. *Br. Med. J.,* **297,** 15–17.

64. Horowitz, M., Need, A. G., Philcox, J. C. and Nordin, B. E. C. (1984). Effect of calcium supplementation on urinary hydroxyproline in osteoporotic postmenopausal women. *Am. J. Clin. Nutr.,* **39,** 857–9.

65. Nordin, B. E. C., Horsman, A., Crilly, R. G., Marshall, D. H. and Simpson, M. (1980). Treatment of spinal osteoporosis in postmenopausal women. *Br. Med. J.,* **280,** 451–4.

66. Recker, R. R., Saville, P. D. and Heaney, R. P. (1977). Effect of estrogens and calcium carbonate on bone loss in postmenopausal women. *Ann. Intern. Med.,* **87,** 649–55.

67. Riis, B., Thomsen, K. and Christiansen, C. (1987). Does calcium supplementation prevent postmenopausal bone loss? A double blind controlled study. *N. Engl. J. Med.,* **316,** 173–7.

68. Lau, E., Donnan, S., Barker, D. J. P. and Cooper, C. (1988). Physical activity and calcium intake in fracture of the proximal femur in Hong Kong. *Br. Med. J.,* **297,** 1441–3.

69. Bernstein, D. S., Sadowsky, N., Hegsted, D. M., Guri, C. D. and Stave, F. J. (1966). Prevalence of osteoporosis in high- and low-fluoride areas in North Dakota. *J. Am. Med. Assoc.,* **198,** 499–504.

70. Alffram, P. A., Hernborg, J. and Nilsson, B. E. R. (1969). The influence of a high fluoride content in the drinking water on the bone mineral mass in man. *Acta. Orthop. Scand.,* **40,** 137–42.

71. Simonen, O. and Laitinen, O. (1985). Does fluoridation of drinking-water prevent bone fragility and osteoporosis? *Lancet,* **2,** 432–3.

72. Heaney, R. P. and Recker, R. R. (1982). Effects of nitrogen, phosphorus, and caffeine on calcium balance in women. *J. Lab. Clin. Med.,* **99,** 46–55.

73. Parfitt, A. M (1983). Dietary risk factors for age-related bone loss and fractures. *Lancet,* **2,** 1181–5.

74. Garn, S. M. and Kangas, J. (1981). Protein intake, bone mass and bone loss. In De Luca, H. F., Frost, H. M., Jee, W. S. S., Johnston, C. C. Jr and Parfitt, A. M. (eds), *Osteoporosis: Recent Advances in Pathogenesis and Treatment* (Baltimore: University Park Press), pp. 257–63.

75. Rigotti, N. A., Nussbaum, S. R., Herzog, D. B. and Neer, R. M. (1984). Osteoporosis in women with anorexia nervosa. *N. Engl. J. Med.,* **311,** 1601–6.

76. Goulding, A. (1980). Effects of dietary NaCl supplements on parathyroid function, bone turnover and bone composition in rats taking restricted amounts of calcium. *Miner. Electrolyte Metab.,* **4,** 203–8.

77. Goulding, A. (1981). Fasting urinary sodium/creatinine in relation to calcium/creatinine and hydroxyproline/creatinine in a general population of women. *NZ Med. J.,* **93,** 294–7.

78. Davidson, B. J., Ross, R. K., Paganini-Hill, A., Hammond, G. D., Siiteri, P. K. and Judd, H. L. (1982). Total and free estrogens and androgens in postmenopausal women with hip fractures. *J. Clin. Endocrinol. Metab.,* **54,** 115–20.

79. Saville, P. D. and Nilsson, B. E. R. (1966). Height and weight in symptomatic postmenopausal osteoporosis. *Clin. Orthop.,* **45,** 49–54.

80. Christiansen, C., Riis, B. J. and Rødbro, P. (1987). Prediction of rapid bone loss in postmenopausal women. *Lancet,* **1,** 1105–8.

81. Frumar, A. M., Meldrum, D. R., Geola, F, Shamonki, I. M., Tataryn, I. V., Deftos, L. J. and Judd, H. L. (1980). Relationship of fasting urinary calcium to circulating estrogen and body weight in postmenopausal women. *J. Clin. Endocrinol. Metab.,* **50,** 70–5.

82. Saville, P. D. (1965). Changes in bone mass with age and alcoholism. *J. Bone Jt. Surg.,* **47A,** 492–9.

83. Bikle, D. D., Genant, H. K., Cann, C., Recker, R. R., Halloran, B. P. and Strewler, G. J. (1985). Bone disease in alcohol abuse. *Ann. Intern. Med.,* **103,** 42–8.

84. Nordin, B. E. C. and Polley, K. J. (1987). Metabolic consequences of the menopause. *Calcif. Tissue Int.,* **41** (Suppl. 1), 1–59.

85. Daniell, H. W. (1976). Osteoporosis of the slender smoker: vertebral compression fractures and loss of metacarpal cortex in relation to postmenopausal cigarette smoking and lack of obesity. *Arch. Intern. Med.,* **136,** 298–304.

86. De Vernejoul, M. C., Bielakoff, J., Herve, M., Gueris, J., Hott, M., Modrowski, D., Kuntz, D., Miravet, L. and Ryckewaert, A. (1983). Evidence for defective osteoblastic function. A role for alcohol and tobacco consumption in osteoporosis in middle-aged men. *Clin. Orthop.,* **179,** 107–15.

87. Jick, H., Porter, J. and Morrison, A. S. (1977). Relation between smoking and the age of natural menopause. *Lancet,* **1,** 1354–5.

88. Jensen, J., Christiansen, C. and Rødbro, P. (1985). Cigarette smoking, serum estrogens and bone loss during hormone-replacement therapy early after menopause. *N. Engl. J. Med.,* **313,** 973–5.

89. Raisz, L. G. (1988). Local and systemic factors in the pathogenesis of osteoporosis. *N. Engl. J. Med.,* **318,** 818–28.

90. Krølner, B., Toft, B., Pors Nielsen, S. and Tøndevold, E. (1983). Physical exercise as prophylaxis against involutional bone loss: a controlled trial. *Clin. Sci.,* **64,** 541–6.

91. Krølner, B. and Toft, B. (1983). Vertebral bone loss: an unheeded effect of therapeutic bed rest. *Clin. Sci.,* **64,** 537–40.

92. Boyce, W. J. and Vessey, M. P. (1988). Habitual physical inertia and other factors in relation to risk of fracture of the proximal femur. *Age Ageing*, **17**, 319–27.

93. Bullamore, J. R., Gallagher, J. C., Wilkinson, R., Nordin, B. E. C. and Marshall, D. H. (1970). Effect of age on calcium absorption. *Lancet*, **2**, 535–7.

94. Wasserman, R. H. (1981). Intestinal absorption of calcium and phosphorus. *Fed. Proc.*, **40**, 68–72.

95. Baker, M. R., Peacock, M. and Nordin, B. E. C. (1980). The decline in vitamin D status with age. *Age Ageing*, **9**, 249–52.

96. Holick, M. F., MacLaughlin, J. A., Clark, M. B., Holick, S. A., Potts, J. T. Jr., Anderson, R. R., Blank, I. H., Parrish, J. A. and Elias, P. (1980). Photosynthesis of previtamin D_3 in human skin and the physiologic consequences. *Science*, **210**, 203–5.

97. Poskitt, E. M. E., Cole, T. J. and Lawson, D. E. M. (1979). Diet, sunlight and 25 hydroxyvitamin D in healthy children and adults. *Br. Med. J.*, **1**, 221–3.

98. Lawson, D. E. M., Paul, A. A., Black, A. E., Cole, T. J., Mandal, A. R. and Davie, M. (1979). Relative contributions of diet and sunlight to vitamin D state in the elderly. *Br. Med. J.*, **2**, 303–5.

99. Barragry, J. M., France, M. W., Corless, D., Gupta, S. P., Switala, S., Boucher, B. J. and Cohen, R. D. (1978). Intestinal cholecalciferol absorption in the elderly and in younger adults. *Clin. Sci.*, **55**, 213–20.

100. Skinner, R. K. (1979). 25 hydroxylation of vitamin D in the elderly. In Norman, A. W., Schaefer, K., Herrath, D. v., Grigoleit, H.-G., Coburn, J. W., DeLuca, H. F., Mawer, E. B. and Suda, T. (eds), *Vitamin D: Basic Research and its Clinical Application* (Berlin, New York: Walter de Gruyter), pp. 1011–13.

101. Fraser, D. R. and Kodicek, E. (1970). Unique biosynthesis by kidney of biologically active vitamin D metabolite. *Nature*, **228**, 764–6.

102. Kodicek, E., Lawson, D. E. M. and Wilson, P. W. (1970). Biological activity of polar metabolite of vitamin D_3. *Nature*, **228**, 763–4.

103. Haussler, M. R. and McCain, T. A. (1977). Basic and clinical concepts related to vitamin D metabolism and action. *N. Engl. J. Med.*, **297**, 974–83, 1041–50.

104. Davies, D. F. and Shock, N. W. (1950). Age changes in glomerular filtration rate, effective renal plasma flow and tubular excretory capacity in adult males. *J. Clin. Invest.*, **29**, 496–507.

105. Francis, R. M., Peacock, M., Storer, J. H., Davies, A. E. J., Brown, W. B. and Nordin, B. E. C. (1983). Calcium malabsorption in the elderly: the effect of treatment with oral 25-hydroxyvitamin D_3. *Eur. J. Clin. Invest.*, **13**, 391–6.

106. Corless, D., Beer, M., Boucher, B. J., Gupta, S. P. and Cohen, R. D. (1975). Vitamin D status in long stay geriatric patients. *Lancet*, **2**, 1404–6.

107. Nayal, A. S., MacLennan, W. J., Hamilton, J. C., Rose, P. and Kong, M. (1978). 25 Hydroxyvitamin D, diet and sunlight exposure in patients admitted to a geriatric unit. *Gerontology*, **24**, 117–22.

108. Francis, R. M., Peacock, M., Taylor, G. A., Storer, J. H. and Nordin, B. E. C. (1984). Calcium malabsorption in elderly women with vertebral fractures: evidence for resistance to the action of vitamin D metabolites on the bowel. *Clin. Sci.*, **66**, 103–7.

109. Francis, R. M., Peacock, M. and Barkworth, S. A. (1984). Renal impairment and its effects on calcium metabolism in elderly women. *Age Ageing*, **13**, 14–20.

110. Cockcroft, D. W. and Gault, M. H. (1976). Prediction of creatinine clearance from serum creatinine. *Nephron, 16*, 31–41.
111. Nordin, B. E. C., Baker, M. R., Horsman, A. and Peacock, M. (1985). A prospective trial of the effect of vitamin D supplementation on metacarpal bone loss in elderly women. *Am. J. Clin. Nutr., 42*, 470–4.
112. Buchanan, J. R., Myers, C. A. and Greer, R. B. III (1988). Effect of declining renal function on bone density in aging women. *Calcif. Tissue Int., 43*, 1–6.
113. Tsai, K.-S., Heath, H. III, Kumar, R. and Riggs, B. L. (1984). Impaired vitamin D metabolism with aging in women: possible role in pathogenesis of senile osteoporosis. *J. Clin. Invest., 73*, 1668–72.
114. Riggs, B. L. and Melton, L. J. III (1983). Evidence for two distinct syndromes of involutional osteoporosis. *Am. J. Med., 75*, 899–901.
115. Peacock, M., Francis, R. M. and Selby, P. L. (1983). Vitamin D and osteoporosis. In Dixon, A. St J., Russell, R. G. G. and Stamp, T. C. B. (eds), *Osteoporosis: A Multidisciplinary Problem* (London: Academic Press), pp. 245–54.
116. Marshall, D. H., Crilly, R. G. and Nordin, B. E. C. (1977). Plasma androstenedione and oestrone levels in normal and osteoporotic postmenopausal women. *Br. Med. J., 2*, 1177–9.
117. Gallagher, J. C., Riggs, B. L., Eisman, J., Hamstra, A., Arnaud, S. B. and DeLuca, H. F. (1979). Intestinal calcium absorption and serum vitamin D metabolites in normal subjects and osteoporotic patients. Effect of age and dietary calcium. *J. Clin. Invest., 64*, 729–36.
118. Gallagher, J. C., Aaron, J., Horsman, A., Marshall, D. H., Wilkinson, R. and Nordin, B. E. C. (1973). The crush fracture syndrome in postmenopausal women. *Clin. Endocrinol. Metab., 2*, 293–315.
119. Nordin, B. E. C., Peacock, M., Crilly, R. G., Francis, R. M., Speed, R. and Barkworth, S. A. (1981). Summation of risk factors in osteoporosis. In DeLuca, H. F., Jee, W. S. S., Johnston, C. C. Jr and Parfitt, A. M. (eds), *Osteoporosis – Recent Advances in Pathogenesis and Treatment* (Baltimore: University Park Press), pp. 359–67.
120. Slovik, D. M., Adams, J. S., Neer, R. M., Holick, M. F. and Potts, J. T. Jr. (1981). Deficient production of 1,25 dihydroxyvitamin D in elderly osteoporotic patients. *N. Engl. J. Med., 305*, 372–4.
121. Riggs, B. L., Hamstra, A. and DeLuca, H. F. (1981). Assessment of 25 hydroxyvitamin D 1α hydroxylase reserve in postmenopausal osteoporosis by administration of parathyroid extract. *J. Clin. Endocrinol. Metab., 53*, 833–5.
122. Nordin, B. E. C., Peacock, M., Crilly, R. G. and Marshall, D. H. (1979). Calcium absorption and plasma 1,25$(OH)_2$D levels in post-menopausal osteoporosis. In Norman, A. W., Schaefer, K., Herrath, D. v., Grigoleit, H.-G., Coburn, J. W., DeLuca, H. F., Mawer, E. B. and Suda, T. (eds), *Vitamin D: Basic Research and its Clinical Application* (Berlin, New York: Walter de Gruyter), pp. 99–106.
123. Jackson, J. A., Kleerekoper, M., Parfitt, A. M., Rao, D. S., Villaneuva, A. R. and Frame, B. (1987). Bone histomorphometry in hypogonadal and eugonadal men with spinal osteoporosis. *J. Clin. Endocrinol. Metab., 65*, 53–8.
124. Eisenhardt, L. and Thompson, K. W. (1939). Brief consideration of present status of so-called basophilism with a tabulation of verified cases. *Yale J. Biol. Med., 11*, 507–22.
125. Kimberg, D. V. (1969). Effects of vitamin D and steroid hormones on the active transport of calcium by the intestine. *N. Engl. J. Med., 280*, 1396–1405.

126. Fucik, R. F., Kukreja, S. C., Hargis, G. K., Bowser, E. N., Henderson, W. J. and Williams, G. A. (1975). Effect of glucocorticoids on function of the parathyroid glands in man. *J. Clin. Endocrinol. Metab.*, **40**, 152–5.

127. Hahn, T. J., Halstead, L. R. and Baran, D. T. (1981). Effects of short-term corticosteroid administration on intestinal calcium absorption and circulating vitamin D metabolite concentrations in man. *J. Clin. Endocrinol. Metab.*, **52**, 111–15.

128. Crilly, R. G., Marshall, D. H. and Nordin, B. E. C. (1979). Metabolic effects of corticosteroid therapy in postmenopausal women. *J. Steroid Biochem.*, **11**, 429–3.

129. Bar-Shavit, Z., Kahn, A. J., Pegg, L. E., Stone, K. R. and Teitelbaum, S. L. (1984). Glucocorticoids modulate macrophage surface oligosaccharides and their bone binding activity. *J. Clin. Invest.*, **73**, 1277–83.

130. Bar-Shavit, Z., Teitelbaum, S. L. and Kahn, A. J. (1983). Saccharides mediate the attachment of rat macrophages to bone in vitro. *J. Clin. Invest.*, **72**, 516–25.

131. Hall, D. H. (1977). Synergistic effect of age and corticosteroid treatment on connective tissue metabolism. *Ann. Rheum. Dis.*, **36s**, 58–62.

132. Mundy, G. R., Raisz, L. G., Cooper, R. A., Schechter, G. P. and Salmon, S. E. (1974). Evidence for the secretion of an osteoclast stimulating factor in myeloma. *N. Engl. J. Med.*, **291**, 1041–6.

133. Garrett, I. R., Durie, B. G. M., Nedwin, G. E., Gillespie, A., Bringman, T., Sabatini, M., Bertolini, D. R. and Mundy, G. R. (1987). Production of lymphotoxin, a bone-resorbing cytokine, by cultured human myeloma cells. *N. Engl. J. Med.*, **317**, 526–32.

134. Krane, S. M. and Schiller, A. L. (1987). Hyperostosis, neoplasms, and other disorders of bone and cartilage. In Braunwald, E., Isselbacher, K. J., Petersdorf, R. G., Wilson, J. D., Martin, J. B. and Fauci, A. S. (eds), *Harrison's Principles of Internal Medicine*, 11th edn (New York: McGraw-Hill), pp. 1902–10.

135. Galasko, C. S. B. (1976). Mechanisms of bone destruction in the development of skeletal metastases. *Nature*, **263**, 507–8.

136. Eilon, G. and Mundy, G. R. (1978). Direct resorption of bone by human breast cancer cells in vitro. *Nature*, **276**, 726–8.

137. Francis, R. M., Perry, H. M., Dunn, J., Kahn, A. J. and Teitelbaum, S. L. (1985). The stimulation of bone resorption by human breast cancer cell lines. *Clin. Sci.*, **68**, 19 p.

138. Koutsilleris, M., Rabbani, S. A., Bennett, H. P. J. and Goltzman, D. (1987). Characteristics of prostate-derived growth factors for cells of the osteoblast phenotype. *J. Clin. Invest.*, **80**, 941–6.

139. Hordon, L. H., Francis, R. M., Marshall, D. H., Smith, A. H. and Peacock, M. (1986). Are scintigrams of the spine useful in vertebral osteoporosis? *Clin. Radiol.*, **37**, 487–9.

140. Hahn, T. J. (1980). Drug-induced disorders of vitamin D and mineral metabolism. *Clin. Endocrinol. Metab.*, **9**, 107–29.

141. Adams, P. H., Jowsey, J., Kelly, P. J., Riggs, B. L., Kinney, V. R. and Jones, J. D. (1967). Effect of hyperthyroidism on bone and mineral metabolism. *Q. J. Med.*, **36**, 1–15.

142. Francis, R. M., Barnett, M. J., Selby, P. L. and Peacock, M. (1982). Thyrotoxicosis presenting as fracture of femoral neck. *Br. Med. J.*, **285**, 97–8.

143. Francis, R. M. and Peacock, M. (1987). The pathogenesis of osteoporosis in

thyrotoxicosis. In Christiansen, C., Johansen, J. S. and Riis, B. J. (eds), *Osteoporosis 1987* (Copenhagen: Osteopress ApS), pp. 166–7.

144. Saville, P. D. (1973). The syndrome of spinal osteoporosis. *Clin. Endocrinol. Metab.*, **2**, 177–85.

145. Winks, C. S. and Felts, W. J. L. (1980). Effects of castration on the bone structure of male rats: a model of osteoporosis. *Calcif. Tissue Int.*, **32**, 77–82.

146. Delmas, P. and Meunier, P. J. (1981). L'osteoporose au cours du syndrome de Klinefelter. *Nouv. Presse Med.*, **10**, 687–90.

147. Baran, D. T., Bergfeld, M. A., Teitelbaum, S. L. and Avioli, L. V. (1978). Effect of testosterone therapy on bone formation in an osteoporotic hypogonadal male. *Calcif. Tissue Res.*, **26**, 103–6.

148. Smith, D. A. S. and Walker, M. S. (1977). Changes in plasma steroids and bone density in Klinefelter's syndrome. *Calcif. Tissue Res.*, **22S**, 225–8.

149. Foresta, C., Busnardo, B., Ruzza, G., Zanatta, G. and Mioni, R. (1983). Lower calcitonin levels in young hypogonadic men with osteoporosis. *Horm. Metab. Res.*, **15**, 206–7.

150. Drinkwater, B. L., Nilson, K., Chesnut, C. H. III, Bremner, W. J., Shainholtz, S. and Southworth, M. B. (1984). Bone mineral content of amenorrheic and eumenorrheic athletes. *N. Engl. J. Med.*, **311**, 277–81.

151. Marcus, R., Cann, C., Madvig, P., Minkoff, J., Goddard, M., Bayer, M., Martin, M., Gaudiani, L., Haskell, W. and Genant, H. (1985). Menstrual function and bone mass in elite women distance runners. *Ann. Intern. Med.*, **102**, 158–63.

152. Heath, H. (1985). Athletic women, amenorrhea and skeletal integrity. *Ann. Intern. Med.*, **102**, 258–60.

153. Riggs, B. L. and Eastell, R. (1986). Exercise, hypogonadism and osteopenia. *J. Am. Med. Assoc.*, **256**, 392–3.

154. Nelson, M. E., Fisher, E. C., Catsos, P. D., Meredith, C. N., Turksoy, R. N. and Evans, W. J. (1986). Diet and bone status in amenorrheic runners. *Am. J. Clin. Nutr.*, **43**, 910–16.

155. Frisch, R. E., Gotz-Welbergen, A. V., McArthur, J. W., Albright, T., Witschi, J., Bullen, B., Birnholz, J., Reed, R. B. and Hermann, H. (1981). Delayed menarche and amenorrhea of college athletes in relation to age of onset of training. *J. Am. Med. Assoc.*, **246**, 1559–63.

156. Drinkwater, B. L., Nilson, K., Ott, S. and Chesnut, C. H. III (1986). Bone mineral density after resumption of menses in amenorrheic athletes. *J. Am. Med. Assoc.*, **256**, 380–2.

157. Szmukler, G. I., Brown, S. W., Parsons, V. and Darby, A. (1985). Premature loss of bone in chronic anorexia nervosa. *Br. Med. J.*, **290**, 26–7.

158. Treasure, J. L., Russell, G. F. M., Fogelman, I. and Murby, B. (1987). Reversible bone loss in anorexia nervosa. *Br. Med. J.*, **295**, 474–5.

159. Bachmann, G. A. and Kemmann, E. (1982). Prevalence of oligomenorrhea and amenorrhea in a college population. *Am. J. Obstet. Gynecol.*, **144**, 98–102.

160. Klibanski, A., Neer, R. M., Beitins, I. Z., Ridgway, E. C., Zervas, N. T. and McArthur, J. W. (1980). Decreased bone density in hyperprolactinemic women. *N. Engl. J. Med.*, **303**, 1511–14.

161. Cann, C. E., Martin, M. C., Genant, H. K. and Jaffe, R. B. (1984). Decreased spinal mineral content in amenorrheic women. *J. Am. Med. Assoc.*, **251**, 626–9.

162. Jackson, J. A., Kleerekoper, M. and Parfitt, A. M. (1986). Symptomatic osteo-

porosis in a man with hyperprolactinemic hypogonadism. *Ann. Intern. Med.,* **105,** 543–5.

163. Greenspan, S. L., Neer, R. M., Ridgway, E. C. and Klibanski, A. (1986). Osteoporosis in men with hyperprolactinemic hypogonadism. *Ann. Intern. Med.,* **104,** 777–82.

164. Klibanski, A. and Greenspan, S. L. (1986). Increase in bone mass after treatment of hyperprolactinemic amenorrhea. *N. Engl. J. Med.,* **315,** 542–6.

165. Selby, P. L. (1988). Osteopenia and diabetes. *Diabetic Med.,* **5,** 423–8.

166. Farley, J. R., Fitzsimmons, R., Taylor, A. K., Jorch, U. M. and Lau K.-H. W. (1985). Direct effects of ethanol on bone resorption and formation in vitro. *Arch. Biochem. Biophys.* **238,** 305–14.

167. Spencer, H., Rubio, N., Rubio, E., Indreika, M. and Seitam, A. (1986). Chronic alcoholism. Frequently overlooked cause of osteoporosis in men. *Am. J. Med.,* **80,** 393–7.

168. Lindsell, D. R. M., Wilson, A. G. and Maxwell, J. D. (1982). Fractures on chest radiograph in detection of alcoholic liver disease. *Br. Med. J.,* **285,** 597–9.

169. Minaire, P., Meunier, P., Edouard, C., Bernard, J., Courpron, P. and Bourret, J. (1974). Quantitative histological data on disuse osteoporosis. *Calcif. Tissue Res.,* **17,** 57–73.

170. Anon (1983). Osteoporosis and activity. *Lancet,* **1,** 1365–6.

171. Mazess, R. B. and Whedon, G. D. (1983). Immobilization and bone. *Calcif. Tissue Int.,* **35,** 265–7.

172. Woolf, A. D. and Dixon, A. St. J. (1988). *Osteoporosis: a clinical guide* (London: Martin Dunitz).

173. Bowley, N. B. (1984). Various osteopathies. In Nordin, B. E. C. (ed.), *Metabolic Bone and Stone Disease,* 2nd edn (Edinburgh, London, Melbourne, New York: Churchill Livingstone), pp. 234–7.

174. Mudd, S. H. and Levy, H. L. (1983). Disorders of transsulfuration. In Stanbury, J. B., Wyngaarden, J. B., Fredrickson, D. S., Goldstein, J. L. and Brown, M. S. (eds), *The Metabolic Basis of Inherited Disease,* 5th edn (New York: McGraw Hill), pp. 522–59.

175. Brenton, D. P., Dow, C. J., James, J. I. P., Hay, R. L. and Wynne-Davies, R. (1972). Homocystinuria and Marfan's syndrome. A comparison. *J. Bone Jt. Surg.,* **54B,** 277–98.

176. Dehnel, J. M. and Francis, M. J. O. (1972). Somatomedin (sulphation factor)-like activity of homocystine. *Clin. Sci.,* **43,** 903–6.

4

OESTROGEN AND BONE

P. L. SELBY

INTRODUCTION

In 1941 Fuller Albright described a group of 42 patients with osteo-porosis; of the subjects in his report all but five were postmenopausal women[1]. Since those five patients were all thyrotoxic, and hence had a perfectly adequate explanation for their osteoporosis in any case, this observation led to the suggestion that the menopause might be an important risk factor for osteoporosis. Subsequent observations by the same group confirmed that these results were correct, and that there is an accelerated rate of bone loss after the menopause in normal, as well as osteoporotic, women[2]. The very rapid nature of this loss means that it is one of the most important determinants of bone mass in the postmenopausal woman, and hence a major risk factor for the increased rate of fracture seen in such women. Clearly, an under-standing of the mechanisms by which oestrogen acts upon bone might be of great benefit for the planning of appropriate therapeutic regimens to reduce postmenopausal bone loss, and with it the increased fracture incidence. Unfortunately, until very recently there has been no con-sensus as to this mechanism, and even now many doubts as to its true nature remain. This chapter seeks to review the effects of oestrogen upon bone and the means by which these might be brought about.

MENOPAUSE AND BONE MASS

The observations of Albright had suggested that oestrogen had an important effect in the preservation of bone mass, and were supported by postmortem studies in which the actual mass of individual bones could be measured directly. However the earliest *in vivo* observations of the effect of the menopause upon bone mass were not conclusive[3]. This was because the only means of such measurement available was by densitometry from radiographs, which is very insensitive, and it was not until the advent of more sophisticated techniques that the bone changes associated with the menopause could be detected.

Some of the earliest information about these changes was obtained by morphometric measurements of cortical bones on plain radiographs. The results of many of the early investigations of this type were reviewed by Newton-John and Morgan when they were developing their hypothesis linking bone mass with fracture incidence[4]. In general, the studies indicate a gradual loss of bone with age in both sexes, with a marked acceleration in the rate of loss at, or about, the time of menopause in women. Although these initial studies were usually based on cross-sectional measurements in a population similar results have also been obtained by later, longitudinal, studies[5,6]. At about the same time similar techniques were being applied to matched groups of pre- and postmenopausal women, and a significant bone deficit shown in the latter compared with the former[7].

Such morphometric studies are unable to give any information as to the changes that may or may not be occurring in trabecular bone. Bone volume measurements on iliac crest biopsies would suggest that the changes are similar to those which occur in the cortex[8], but it has only been with the advent of non-invasive techniques for the estimation of trabecular bone mass that large-scale studies on the change in trabecular bone at the time of the menopause could be undertaken. It is now evident that, if anything, the changes in trabecular bone mass which occur in conjunction with the menopause are even more marked than those that occur in cortical bone[9].

So great is the importance of the menopause in determining bone mass that, in postmenopausal women, years since menopause is usually a better predictor of bone mass than is chronological age[10-12]. However, there are several different changes that take place at, or near, the age of menopause. The most obvious of these is the very marked fall in plasma oestrogen concentrations which is the hallmark of the climacteric but there is, in addition, a concomitant rise in gonadotrophins, an absence of the usual monthly surge of progesterone and, shortly afterwards, a fall in androgen levels. Although any or all of these could theoretically influence bone turnover, the two most likely candidates for this role are the changing levels of oestrogens and androgens in the plasma. That the observed change is due to the fall in plasma oestrogen concentration is seen in several studies of perimenopausal women where bone mass relates much more closely to measured oestrogen status than to that of androgens or other menopausal changes[12-14].

OTHER LOW OESTROGEN STATES AND BONE MASS

It has been known for several years that conditions which result in chronic low oestrogen levels, such as Turner's syndrome or other forms of gonadal dysgenesis, lead to an increased risk of osteoporosis[15]. More recently it has been discovered that bone mass is reduced by shorter periods of poor oestrogenization. Perhaps the most common condition causing this is hyperprolactinaemia, which has now been shown to be associated with decreased bone mass by a variety of different investigators[16-20]. Two more recent studies have shown that, in contrast to amenorrhoeic patients, women with hyperprolactinaemia and normal menstruation have normal bone density[21,22]. Since the two patient groups differed only in their oestrogen status, and not in prolactin concentration or other possible confounding variables, this observation underlines the importance of oestrogen for the preservation of bone mass. Treatment of the hyperprolactinaemia by either adenomectomy or bromocriptine results in normalization of oestrogen status and regaining at least some of the lost bone[20].

Similar bone loss is also seen in amenorrhoeic patients with anorexia nervosa[23,24], and in high-performance female athletes who train to such a level as to induce amenorrhoea[25,26]. This last observation is particularly interesting, since it is known that under other circumstances physical exercise is beneficial to the skeleton. Once again, this serves to demonstrate the central and, perhaps predominant, role played by oestrogen in the maintenance of skeletal integrity.

It is now possible to induce a temporary 'artificial menopause' in women by the use of the long-acting LHRH analogues; buserilin, goserilin and nafarelin, which are under investigation for the therapy of a variety of benign conditions including endometriosis, dysmenorrhoea and dysfunctional uterine bleeding, in addition to their well-established role in the treatment of malignancy. During such treatment it has been shown that there is a rapid loss of bone, and that this is largely, if not completely, replaced on cessation of therapy when the oestrogen levels return to normal[27,28].

Oestrogen treatment and bone mass

Long before it was realized that these potentially reversible low-oestrogen states could result in temporary bone loss, which abated with the restoration of plasma oestrogen to normal, it was reasoned that, if oestrogen deficiency lay at the root of postmenopausal bone loss, then oestrogen replacement might be a useful preventive treatment. Although such therapy had been shown to have a beneficial effect on both direct and indirect measures of bone turnover (see below)[2,29-33], it was not until modern techniques for estimating bone mass were introduced that a beneficial effect of postmenopausal oestrogen replacement on skeletal mass was observed directly. Since then this observation has been confirmed on numerous occasions using a variety of different techniques of estimating bone density at both cortical and trabecular sites[34-40]. It is now clear that the action on bone is independent of the type of oestrogen given or the route of delivery. It is dose-dependent with a plasma oestradiol concentration of 150–200 pmol/l necessary to prevent bone loss after percutaneous administration[41,42] or a daily dose in excess of 15 μg of ethinyloestradiol[43] or of 0.625 mg of conjugated equine oestrogens[44-46].

There has now been sufficient long-term experience with postmenopausal oestrogen administration to demonstrate that, in addition to preserving bone mass, it does indeed reduce the risk of subsequent fracture. This was first suggested by the work of Wallach and Henneman, who suggested that the preservation of height in osteoporotic women receiving oestrogen was the result of the prevention of further vertebral fractures[45]. Further support for the contention that oestrogen reduces vertebral compression fracture prevalence has been given by later studies[46-49]. However, some commentators have cast doubt on these studies, suggesting that they have not been adequately controlled, and that the observed changes in fracture incidence could be related to the natural history of osteoporosis itself[50].

The osteoporotic fracture which is associated with most morbidity and mortality is that of the femoral neck. Accordingly it is not surprising that most attention has been directed towards demonstrating the ability of oestrogen replacement to prevent this fracture. In view of the long latent period between menopause and time of fracture in most women it has not been possible to address this problem by means of a double-blind placebo-controlled trial, instead the information has been derived either from case–control studies of femoral fracture victims or else cohort studies of oestrogen-treated women.

TABLE 4.1 Case–control studies of oestrogen use in patients with femoral fracture

Reference	Number of patients	Number receiving oestrogen	
		Observed	Expected
51	80	8	20
52	320	109	166
53	83	35	43
54	168	49	61
55	94	14	25

Overall $\chi^2 = 35.5$; $p = 4 \times 10^{-7}$.

Several case–control studies have demonstrated that women who have received oestrogen replacement are less likely to sustain a femoral fracture (Table 4.1)[50-55]. More detailed analysis provided by some of these studies suggests that the greatest benefit is provided by prolonged treatment, and that periods of therapy of less than 5 years are of little benefit. In addition, protection is lost with the passage of time after the cessation of therapy.

Only two cohort studies of fracture incidence in patients receiving oestrogen have as yet been reported (Table 4.2). The first of these was a relatively small study in fairly young women, and failed to show any benefit whatsoever on femoral fracture incidence[49]; it did, however, demonstrate a marked reduction in the incidence of other osteoporotic fractures in women receiving oestrogen. The other study was part of the Framingham study and, as such, was considerably larger; in addition, the patients were appreciably older. In this instance a reduction of femoral fracture incidence of about 35% was seen in the oestrogen-treated group[56].

TABLE 4.2   Cohort studies of femoral fracture incidence in women receiving oestrogen

Reference	Patient-years of oestrogen	Number of fractures	
		Observed	Expected
49	4,312	2	2*
56	11,102	28	41

* Significant differences at other fracture sites

It is therefore abundantly clear that postmenopausal oestrogen replacement is of benefit to the skeleton. Unfortunately hormone replacement therapy is not universally acceptable; some women have contraindications to its use, although such instances are becoming less common with the increased understanding of the pharmacology of oestrogen replacement that underlies the newer hormone replacement regimens. More important is the fact that a lot of women are not prepared to accept long-term oestrogen therapy, especially since, in the majority of instances, this will necessitate the continuation or even resumption of menstruation[57]. This poses a particular problem in women who do not suffer from symptoms of the climacteric, but who have been recommended to take oestrogen for the sake of the skeleton: these are precisely those women in whom we should want to encourage prolonged hormone replacement therapy. If the mechanism by which oestrogen acts upon bone could be identified it might allow a therapy with the benefits of oestrogen, but without its drawbacks, to be devised.

MODE OF ACTION OF OESTROGEN UPON BONE

From his early studies of the action of oestrogen in calcium balance studies Albright reached the conclusion that its predominant action was anabolic[2]. Later work has suggested otherwise, and that its predominant action is as an antagonist of bone resorption. The evidence for this is from a variety of different sources. In the first place, oestrogen treatment causes a reduction in markers of bone turnover, not only urinary excretion of calcium and hydroxyproline[29-33] which indicate the rate of resorption, but also plasma alkaline phosphatase activity[29] and osteocalcin concentration[58] which reflect bone formation. This observation is completely contrary to those which would have been predicted by Albright's hypothesis, namely an increase in the plasma osteocalcin concentration and alkaline phosphatase activity. Further evidence that the action of oestrogen is predominantly anti-catabolic is given by bone turnover measurements made with radio-isotopes during calcium balance studies[31,32]. These show quite marked suppression of both bone formation and resorption during oestrogen treatment. Similar results are also obtained from the studies of bone histomorphometry[33] or by microradiographic studies[29] of bone biopsies. In addition, studies of the morphometry of the metacarpals on sequential radiographs taken during the course of oestrogen therapy demonstrate an inhibition of bone resorption which takes place at the endosteal surface whilst bone formation at the periosteum continues unaltered[43].

MECHANISM OF ACTION OF OESTROGEN UPON BONE

Although it is now clear that oestrogen is primarily an inhibitor of bone resorption, the mechanism by which it brings about this action is even now not clear. Two early studies suggested that there was a direct effect of oestrogen to inhibit bone resorption induced by parathyroid hormone or vitamin D metabolites *in vitro*[59,60]. However, others demonstrated that this was a non-specific toxic effect of the unphysiological doses of oestrogen used, and that analogous results could be obtained using the inactive sterol 17α-oestradiol, or even the steroid precursor, cholesterol[61,62]. In all other target issues for

87

oestrogen there exist specific high-affinity receptor proteins. Until recently it has not been possible to demonstrate such receptors in bone cells[63-66]; although several recent studies have now suggested that such molecules do exist in the skeleton of adults they have only been detected in the osteoblast or bone forming cells[67-69] and not in the bone-resorbing osteoclasts. Furthermore, although those cells in which such receptors have been identified are capable of responding to oestrogen the changes induced by oestrogen are either non-specific effects which occur in all oestrogen-sensitive tissues – for example the induction of progesterone receptors[67], or are specific changes that might be taken to indicate an increase in bone formation, such as the production of procollagen or transforming growth factor[68-70]. These observations make a direct effect of oestrogen upon bone-resorbing cells still appear unlikely.

In view of this apparent lack of oestrogen receptors within osteo-clasts a variety of hypotheses were put forward involving indirect mechanisms whereby oestrogen might act on bone. Although such mechanisms might appear to be largely irrelevant in view of the discovery of oestrogen receptors in bone, this is not the case since, as outlined above, the receptors have not been found in cells directly concerned with bone resorption. Some consideration of these alter-native explanations is therefore necessary for a complete under-standing of the action of oestrogen upon bone.

The earliest explanation to be put forward was advanced inde-pendently by two separate groups in 1965, each suggesting that oestrogen diminished the sensitivity of bone to external bone-resorbing stimuli, most probably parathyroid hormone (PTH)[71,72]. No mech-anism for this was put forward, but the *in vitro* results of Atkins were originally thought to support this concept. Since these latter results have been shown to be artefactual (see above) no convincing alter-native explanation has been put forward. Nevertheless oestrogen is known to have profound effects on cellular behaviour in other systems, and so it is not possible to exclude this hypothesis as the means whereby oestrogen does influence bone. Indeed, since it is known that the action of PTH on bone resorption is not due to a direct effect on osteoclasts but is mediated by an as yet ill-defined paracrine mech-anism involving PTH receptors on osteoblasts[73,74] it might even be that the recent discovery of oestrogen receptors in these cells is suggestive of the operation of just such a mechanism. Set against this must be the failure of the majority of investigators to demonstrate any action of oestrogen on PTH-induced bone resorption *in vitro*[61,62] when the other actions of osteoclasts, which are apparently mediated by a paracrine influence of oesteoblasts, are readily demonstrable in tissue culture[74,75].

In addition to such a direct action of oestrogen to reduce bone resorption at least two further more indirect mechanisms have been put forward whereby it might influence bone. Each of these involves changes in the calcium-regulating hormones and their actions: one suggesting that oestrogen administration stimulates calcitonin production, thereby protecting bone; the other that oestrogen administration increases the absorption of calcium from the gastrointestinal tract, this reducing the need of the body to draw on skeletal calcium for homeostatic purposes.

The calcitonin hypothesis

Calcitonin is a powerful inhibitor of bone resorption in pharmacological doses, and may even exert this action at physiological concentrations[76]. Calcitonin concentrations are lower in women than men[77,78] and some, but by no means all, observers have suggested a fall in calcitonin concentrations at the time of the menopause[79,80]. Taking these observations with *in vitro* studies which suggest an effect of oestrogen on calcitonin secretion[81,82] it is not surprising that this hormone has been identified as a candidate whereby oestrogen could act indirectly on bone. This speculation was furthered by the observation that calcitonin response to calcium infusion was blunted in postmenopausal women but restored to normal by oestrogen administration[83], and that oestrogen administration increased midday fasting plasma calcitonin concentrations after the menopause[84]. However, these results have not been capable of reproduction by other groups[85,86] and, in particular, using a rather elegant technique of the 'calcium clamp' Torring has been unable to demonstrate any difference in calcitonin secretion, either basal or following calcium stimulation, between pre- and postmenopausal women[87,88]. Indeed he was unable to demonstrate any influence of oestrogen status on calcitonin secretion. Although calcitonin in pharmacological doses may be of benefit in the management of some patients with osteoporosis (Chapter 6), there is little evidence that calcitonin deficiency in man is associated with excessive bone loss. One study of patients post-total thyroidectomy, and hence presumably calcitonin-deficient, did reveal a deficit of forearm bone mineral, but this could easily be explicable in terms of the larger doses of exogenous thyroxine taken by the patients under study compared with the control subjects[89]. Conversely, another study which examined bone density in a group of patients with documented calcitonin deficiency following subtotal thyroidectomy was unable to demonstrate such a difference[90]. Perhaps the most telling evidence against the 'calcitonin hypothesis' of oestrogen's action on bone is obtained from studies of calcitonin concentrations in patients with osteoporotic fracture. Although two relatively early studies did suggest that plasma calcitonin concentrations are decreased in patients with osteoporotic fractures[91,92] this has not been confirmed by more recent studies, all of which show increased calcitonin concentrations in patients with fractures[93–95]. These latter observations strongly suggest that, far from protecting home, the raised calcitonin is a physiological response to the increased bone resorption which continues unabated.

Calcium absorption hypothesis

Since over 99% of the body's calcium is found in the skeleton this is vulnerable to mobilization to maintain plasma calcium in times of calcium deficiency. It is therefore not surprising that postmenopausal osteoporosis has been suggested to arise as a result of a stress on calcium homeostasis leading to increased bone resorption. The most common cause which is suggested for this stress is a fall in calcium absorption. In support of this hypothesis is the observation that there is a fall in calcium absorptive efficiency at the time of the menopause measurable by calcium balance studies[96], even if this is not reproducible using radiocalcium tracer studies[97]. In addition, many studies have demonstrated that long-term oestrogen therapy leads to an increase in calcium absorption measured by a variety of different means including radiocalcium studies[96,98–100]. A variety of studies have suggested that the reason underlying the change in calcium absorption is an oestrogen-stimulated increase in the production of the active metabolite of vitamin D, calcitriol, as a result of enhanced 1α-hydroxy-lase activity in the kidney[99]. Although this enzyme has been shown to be stimulated by oestrogen in birds[101,102] this has not been demonstrated in mammals, and so the relevance of this mechanism in man must be questioned. Nevertheless several authors have demonstrated an apparent rise in plasma calcitriol concentration following oestrogen administration to postmenopausal women. Unfortunately, none of these reports has taken note of the fact that calcitriol is transported in the plasma bound to vitamin D binding protein (DBP)[103], and that in common with other binding proteins DBP concentrations are increased markedly by oral oestrogen administration[104]. If DBP concentrations are measured in addition to those of calcitriol and the free plasma concentration of calcitriol calculated then there is no significant change during oestrogen treatment[86]. The rise in DBP concentration is due to a pharmacological action of oestrogen which, on being absorbed from the gut, passes to the liver in high concentrations, where it provokes the observed changes in binding proteins. If oestrogen is given via a transdermal delivery system no such stimulation of the liver occurs, there is no increase in DBP production and no changes in either plasma calcitriol concentration or calcium absorption take place [105]. Thus, if oestrogen administration does increase calcium absorption it is not by way of increased calcitriol concentration. It has been suggested that oestrogen might increase the number of calcitriol receptors in the intestinal mucosa, and thus increase the efficiency of gastrointestinal calcium absorption in response to any particular concentration of calcitriol, and this remains a possible explanation for the observed effect of oestrogen on calcium absorption[106]. The change in receptor number is not present until after several weeks of oestrogen administration; this is in keeping with the observed increase in calcium absorption which is present after prolonged oestrogen replacement[96,98–100], but not after 3 weeks' therapy[86]. Hence it is impossible to invoke this change in calcium absorption in the antiresorptive action of oestrogen which is complete within 3 weeks of commencing treatment[86]. If bone resorption were increased in order to compensate for falling calcium absorption after the menopause it might be expected that the stimulus for this would be reduced plasma calcium concentrations at the menopause, which would be restored to their premenopausal level by oestrogen therapy.

Precisely the opposite changes occur, indicating this not to be the case[86]. Far more likely is that the observed increase in calcium absorption following oestrogen replacement is a secondary homeostatic response to the fall in plasma calcium as a result of the decreased rate of bone resorption induced by the treatment.

Other endocrine mechanisms

Indirect mechanisms for oestrogen to act on bone via other endocrine systems have been proposed, but have not received general acceptance. One group has postulated an action on the growth hormone–somatomedin system, but this might be expected to act on bone formation and is therefore unable to explain the observed facts[107]. Another group has suggested an action via prostaglandin production but as yet this has only been demonstrated in tissue culture and so its relevance in the intact human is questionable[108].

Effect on osteoclast recruitment

It can therefore be seen that none of the currently accepted hypotheses can adequately explain the known facts surrounding the action of oestrogen upon bone. Is it possible to construct a different hypothesis which will more adequately explain the known facts?

In order to do so it is necessary to look at the time course of the action of oestrogen upon bone. As stated above, its effect on resorption is complete within about 3 weeks, although it takes much longer for bone formation to reach a new steady state. This is probably a passive response resulting from the tight coupling which exists between bone formation and resorption. From this time course it is clear that oestrogen is most unlikely to be having a direct effect on mature osteoclasts. If this were the case a much more rapid inhibition of bone resorption would be expected, as is seen following treatment with calcitonin[109] or bisphosphonates[110]. It is known that bone turnover arises as a result of the concerted action of groups of forming and resorbing cells which together form basic multicellular units (BMU). In the life of any one of these units there is a period of bone resorption followed by a resting phase, after which matrix formation and then mineralization take place. Under normal circumstances the resorptive phase of each of these cycles of BMU activity is of the order of 3 weeks. Hence any compound which inhibited the induction of new resorbing cells might be expected to achieve its maximum effect on bone resorption after 3 weeks, when all the osteoclasts which had already begun to act before treatment was commenced would have completed their cycles of activity. There is already some independent evidence in the literature to support such an explanation for the action of oestrogen on bone, in the form of a histomorphometric study by Frost[33]. More recently little attention has been paid to any possible effect that oestrogen might have on osteoclast differentiation; although it has been mentioned as a possible site of action by some authors they did not discuss any mechanism whereby this might be brought about[111].

Before accepting any such model for the effect of oestrogen upon bone it must be asked if there is any realistic mechanism whereby such an action could be brought about. At least two possible candidates exist: by a direct action on osteoclast precursors; or via the mediation of osteoblasts.

Although there is still some controversy about the precise derivation of osteoclast precursors it is generally accepted that they are derived from a circulating population of mononuclear cells and not, as was previously believed, from tissue macrophages[112]. It is well established that many cells of the mononuclear series possess oestrogen receptors, and that in such cells oestrogen is capable of influencing cell growth and division[113-115]. Thus it is not inconceivable that osteoclast precursors do bear oestrogen receptors. If that is the case it is quite likely that the growth and differentiation of those cells would be under the control of oestrogen. Such a hypothesis would require that the receptors be lost during the process of development, but such a phenomenon is well recognized in other situations. Since osteoclast precursors are not found within bone[112] this explanation would account for the inability to find oestrogen receptor protein in bone-resorbing cells. Since the precise nature of the osteoclast precursor is yet to be established this hypothesis is incapable of being formally tested. It is quite likely that this will soon be remedied, with the growing ability to recognize cell surface markers and to separate cells using such markers. In the meantime it has been demonstrated by a variety of investigators that osteoclasts can differentiate from splenic pulp cultured in the presence of bone, and so it may be possible to examine the effect of oestrogen on osteoclast differentiation using this system[116].

Recent work from Japan has suggested an alternative mechanism for the way in which oestrogen might affect bone-resorbing cells. Using the splenic pulp culture system alluded to above these workers were able to demonstrate that the element of bone that was necessary to promote the differentiation of osteoclasts from the pulp was the presence of viable osteoblasts[117]. Since oestrogen receptors are known to be present in these cells, which are capable of responding to oestrogen by altered growth and activity, it is very tempting to postulate that oestrogen may modulate osteoclast differentiation via this or a closely related mechanism. Once again, it is likely that further confirmation of this hypothesis will need to await identification and isolation of the osteoclast precursor cells.

REFERENCES

1. Albright, F., Smith, P. H. and Richelson, A. M. (1941). Postmenopausal osteoporosis: its clinical features. *J. Am. Med. Assoc.*, **116**, 2465–74.
2. Albright, F. (1947). Hormones and human osteogenesis. *Rec. Prog. Horm. Res.*, **1**, 293–353.
3. Donaldson, I. A. and Nassim, J. R. (1954). The artificial menopause with particular reference to the occurrence of spinal porosis. *Br. Med. J.*, **1**, 1228–1331.
4. Newton-John, H. F. and Morgan, D. B. (1970). The loss of bone with age, osteoporosis, and fractures. *Clin. Orthop.*, **71**, 229–52.
5. Adams, P. H., Davies, G. T. and Sweetnam, P. (1970). Osteoporosis and the effects of ageing on bone mass in elderly men and women. *Q. J. Med.*, **39**, 601–15.
6. Horsman, A. (1976). Bone mass. In Nordin, B. E. C. (ed.), *Calcium Phosphate and Magnesium Metabolism*. (Edinburgh: Churchill Livingstone), pp. 357–404.
7. Meema, H. E. (1965). Menopausal and ageing changes in muscle mass and bone. *J. Bone Jt. Surg.*, **48A**, 1138–44.
8. Meunier, P., Courpron, P., Edouard, C., Bernard, J., Brinquier, J. and Vignon, G. (1973). Physiological senile involution and pathological rarefaction of bone: quantitative and comparative histological data. *Clin. Endocrinol. Metab.*, **2**, 239–56.
9. Mazess, R. B. (1982). On aging bone loss. *Clin. Orthop.*, **165**, 239–52.
10. Lindquist, O., Bengtsson, C. and Hansson, T. (1979). Age at menopause and its relation to osteoporosis. *Maturitas*, **1**, 175–81.

11. Richelson, L. S., Wahner, H. W., Melton, L. J. and Riggs, B. L. (1984). Relative contribution of aging and estrogen deficiency to postmenopausal bone loss. *N. Engl. J. Med.*, **311**, 1273–5.
12. Nilas, L. and Christiansen, C. (1987). Bone mass and its relationship to age and the menopause. *J. Clin. Endocrinol. Metab.*, **65**, 697–702.
13. Johnson, C. C., Hui, S. L., Witt, R. M., Appeldorn, R., Baker, R. S. and Longcope, C. (1985). Early menopausal changes in bone mass and sex steroids. *J. Clin. Endocrinol. Metab.*, **61**, 905–11.
14. Slemenda, C., Hui, S. L., Longcope, C. and Johnson, C. C. (1987). Sex steroids and bone mass. A study of changes about the time of menopause. *J. Clin. Invest.*, **80**, 1261–9.
15. Preger, L., Steinbach, H. L. and Moskovitch, P. (1968). Roentgenographic abnormalities in phenotypic females with gonadal dysgenesis. *Am. J. Roentgenol.*, **104**, 899–910.
16. Klibanski, A., Neer, R. M., Beitins, I. Z., Ridgway, E. C., Zervas, N. T. and McArthur, J. W. (1980). Decreased bone density in hyperprolactinaemic women. *N. Engl. J. Med.*, **303**, 1511–14.
17. Schlecte, J. A., Sherman, B. and Martin, R. (1983). Bone density in amenorrheic women with and without hyperprolactinaemia. *J. Clin. Endocrinol. Metab.*, **56**, 1120–3.
18. Koppelman, M. C., Kurtz, D. W., Morrish, K. A., Bou, E., Susser, J. K., Shapiro, J. R. and Loriaux, D. L. (1984). Vertebral body bone mineral content in hyperprolactinaemic women. *J. Clin. Endocrinol. Metab.*, **59**, 1050–3.
19. Cann, C. E., Martin, W. C., Genant, H. K. and Jaffe, R. B. (1984). Decreased spinal mineral content in amenorrheic women. *J. Am. Med. Assoc.*, **251**, 626–9.
20. Klibanski, A. and Greenspan, S. L. (1986). Increase in bone mass after treatment of hyperprolactinemic amenorrhea. *N. Engl. J. Med.*, **315**, 542–6.
21. Ciccarelli, E., Savino, L., Carlevetto, V., Bertagna, A., Isaia, G. C. and Camanni, I. (1988). Vertebral bone density in non-amenorrhoeic hyper-prolactinaemic women. *Clin. Endocrinol.*, **28**, 1–6.
22. Klibanski, A., Biller, B. K. M., Rosethal, D. I., Schoenfeld, D. A. and Saxe, V. (1988). Effects of prolactin and estrogen deficiency in amenorrheic bone loss. *J. Clin. Endocrinol. Metab.*, **67**, 124–30.
23. Rigotti, N. A., Nussbaum, S. R, Herzog, D. B. and Neer, R. M. (1984). Osteo-porosis in women with anorexia nervosa. *N. Engl. J. Med.*, **311**, 1601–6.
24. Szmukler, G. I., Brown, S. W., Parsons, V. and Darby, A. (1985). Premature loss of bone in chronic anorexia nervosa. *Br. Med. J.*, **290**, 26–7.
25. Drinkwater, B. L., Nilson, K., Chesnut, C. H., Bremner, W. J., Shainholtz, S. and Southworth, M. B. (1984). Bone mineral density of amenorrheic and eumenorrheic athletes. *N. Engl. J. Med.*, **311**, 277–81.
26. Lindberg, J. S., Fears, W. B., Hunt, M. M., Powell, M. R., Boll, D. and Wade, C. E. (1984). Exercise induced amenorrhea and bone density. *Ann. Intern. Med.*, **101**, 647–8.
27. Matta, W. H., Shaw, R. W., Hesp, R. and Katz, D. (1987). Hypogonadism induced by luteinising hormone agonist analogues: effects on bone density in premenopausal women. *Br. Med. J.*, **294**, 1523–4.
28. Johansen, J. S., Riis, B. J., Hassager, C., Moen, M., Jacobson, J. and Christi-ansen, C. (1988). The effect of a gonadotropin releasing hormone agonist analog (Nafarelin) on bone metabolism. *J. Clin. Endocrinol Metab.*, **67**, 701–6.

29. Riggs, B. L., Jowsey, J., Kelly, P. J., Jones, D. J. and Maher, F. T. (1969). Effect of sex hormones on bone in primary osteoporosis. *J. Clin. Invest.*, **48**, 1065–72.

30. Gallagher, J. C. and Nordin, B. E. C. (1975). Effects of oestrogen and progestogen therapy on calcium metabolism in post-menopausal women. *Front. Horm. Res.*, **3**, 150–76.

31. Heaney, R. P., Recker, R. R. and Saville, P. D. (1978). Menopausal changes in bone remodelling. *J. Lab. Clin. Med.*, **92**, 964–70.

32. Nordin, B. E. C., Marshall, D. H., Francis, R. M. and Crilly, R. G. (1981). The effects of sex steroid and corticosteroid hormones on bone. *J. Steroid Biochem.*, **15**, 171–4.

33. Frost, H. M. (1973). *Bone Remodelling and its Relationship to Metabolic Bone Diseases* (Springfield, Illinois: Charles C. Thomas).

34. Aitken, J. M., Hart, D. M. and Lindsay, R. (1973). Oestrogen replacement for the prevention of osteoporosis after oophorectomy. *Br. Med. J.*, **2**, 325–8.

35. Meema, S., Bunker, M. L. and Meema, H. E. (1975). Prevention of post-menopausal osteoporosis by hormone treatment of the menopause. *Can. Med. Assoc. J.*, **99**, 248–51.

36. Horsman, A., Gallagher, J. C., Simpson, M. and Nordin, B. E. C. (1977). Prospective trial of oestrogen and calcium in postmenopausal women. *Br. Med. J.*, **2**, 789–92.

37. Recker, R. R., Saville, P. D. and Heaney, R. P. (1977). Effects of estrogens and calcium carbonate on bone loss in postmenopausal women. *Ann. Intern. Med.*, **87**, 649–55.

38. Christiansen, C., Christensen, M. S., McNair, P., Hagen, C., Stocklund, K. E. and Transbol, I. (1980). Prevention of early postmenopausal bone loss: a controlled study in 315 normal females. *Eur. J. Clin. Invest.*, **10**, 273–9.

39. Genant, H. K., Cann, C. E., Ettinger, B. and Gordan, G. S. (1982). Quantitative computed tomography of the vertebral spongiosa: a sensitive method for detecting early bone loss after oophorectomy. *Ann. Intern. Med.*, **97**, 699–705.

40. Riis, B. J., Thomsen, K., Strom, V. and Christiansen, C. (1987). The effect of percutaneous estradiol and natural progesterone on postmenopausal bone loss. *Am. J. Obstet Gynecol.*, **156**, 61–5.

41. Selby, P. L. and Peacock, M. (1986). The dose dependent response of symptoms, pituitary and bone to transdermal oestrogen in postmenopausal women. *Br. Med. J.*, **293**, 1337–9.

42. MacIntyre, I., Stevenson, J. C., Whitehead, M. I., Wimalawansa, S. J., Banks, L. M. and Healy, M. J. R. (1988). Calcitonin for prevention of postmenopausal bone loss. *Lancet*, **1**, 900–1.

43. Horsman, A., Jones, M., Francis, R. and Nordin, C. (1983). The effect of estrogen dose on postmenopausal bone loss. *N. Engl. J. Med.*, **309**, 1405–7.

44. Genant, H. K., Cann, C. E., Ettinger, B. and Gordan, G. S. (1982). Quantitative computed tomography of the vertebral spongiosa: a sensitive method for detecting early bone loss after oophorectomy. *Ann. Intern. Med.*, **97**, 699–705.

45. Wallach, S. and Henneman, P. H. (1959). Prolonged estrogen therapy in postmenopausal women. *J. Am. Med. Assoc.*, **171**, 1637–42.

46. Hutchinson, T. A., Polansky, S. M. and Feinstein, A. R. (1979). Post-menopausal oestrogens protect against fractures of the hip and distal radius. *Lancet*, **2**, 705–9.

47. Lindsay, R., Hart, D. M., Forrest, C. and Baird, C. (1980). Prevention of spinal

osteoporosis in oophorectomised women. *Lancet*, **2**, 1151–54.

48. Riggs, B. L., Seeman, E., Hodgson, S. F., Taves, D. and O'Fallon, W. M. (1982). Effect of the fluoride/calcium regimen on vertebral fracture occurrence in postmenopausal osteoporosis: comparison with conventional therapy. *N. Engl. J. Med.*, **306**, 446–50.

49. Ettinger, B., Gennant, H. K. and Cann, C. E. (1985). Long term estrogen replacement therapy prevents bone loss and fractures. *Ann. Intern. Med.*, **102**, 319–24.

50. Kanis, J. (1984). Treatment of osteoporotic fracture. *Lancet*, **1**, 27–33.

51. Hutchinson, T. A., Polansky, S. M. and Feinstein, A. R. (1979). Post-menopausal oestrogens protect against fractures of the hip and distal radius. *Lancet*, **2**, 705–9.

52. Weiss, N. S., Ure, C. L., Ballard, J. H., Williams, A. R. and Darling, J. R. (1980). Decreased risk of fracture of the hip and lower forearm with postmenopausal use of estrogen. *N. Engl. J. Med.*, **303**, 1195–8.

53. Paganini-Hill, A., Ross, R. K., Gerkins, V. R., Henderson, B. E., Arthur, M. and Mack, T. M. (1981). Menopausal estrogen therapy and hip fractures. *Ann. Intern. Med.*, **95**, 28–31.

54. Johnson, R. E. and Specht, E. E. (1981). The risk of hip fracture in post-menopausal females with and without estrogen drug exposure. *Am. J. Publ. Health*, **71**, 138–44.

55. Kreiger N., Kelsey, J. L., Helford, T. R. and O'Connor, T. (1982). An epidemiologic study of hip fracture in postmenopausal women. *Am. J. Epidemiol.*, **116**, 141–8.

56. Kiel, D. P., Felson, D. T., Anderson, J. J., Wilson, P. W. F. and Moskovitz, M. A. (1987). Hip fractures and the use of estrogen in postmenopausal women. *N. Engl. J. Med.*, **317**, 1169–74.

57. Jones, M. M., Francis, R. M. and Nordin, B. E. C. (1982). Five year follow up of oestrogen therapy in 94 women. *Maturitas*, **4**, 123–30.

58. Selby, P. L. and Brown, W. B. (1988). Bone Gla protein after oestrogen treatment – dissociation from bone formation. *Bone* (In press).

59. Atkins, D., Zanelli, J., Peacock, M. and Nordin, B. E. C. (1972). The effect of oestrogens on the response of bone to parathyroid hormone in vitro. *J. Endocrinol.*, **54**, 107–17.

60. Atkins, D. and Peacock, M. (1975). A comparison of the effects of the calcitonins, sex steroids and thyroid hormones on the response of bone to parathyroid hormone in tissue culture. *J. Endocrinol.*, **64**, 573–83.

61. Caputo, C. B., Meadows, D. and Raisz, L. G. (1978). Failure of estrogen and androgens to inhibit bone resorption in tissue culture. *Endocrinology*, **98**, 1065–8.

62. Francis, R. M., Peacock, M., Taylor, G. A. and Kahn, A. J. (1985). How do oestrogens modulate bone resorption? In Norman, A. W., Schaefer, K., Grigoleit, H.-G. and Herrath, D.v. (eds), *Vitamin D: Chemical, Biochemical and Clinical Update* (Berlin: Walter de Gruyter), pp. 479–80.

63. Nutik, G. and Cruess, R. L. (1974). Estrogen receptors in bone: an evaluation of the uptake of estrogen into bone cells. *Proc. Soc. Exp. Biol. Med.*, **146**, 265–8.

64. Liskova, M. (1976). Influence of estrogens on bone resorption in organ culture. *Calcif. Tissue Res.*, **22**, 207–18.

65. Van Paasen, H. C, Poortman, J., Bogart-Creutzburg, J. H. H. and Duursma,

S. A. (1978). Oestrogen binding proteins in bone cell cytosol. *Calcif. Tissue Res.*, **25**, 249–54.

66. Chen, T. L. and Feldman, D. (1978). Distinction between alfa-fetoprotein and intracellular estrogen receptors: evidence against the presence of estradiol receptors in rat bone. *Endocrinology*, **102**, 236–44.

67. Eriksen, E. F., Colvard, D. S., Berg, N. J., Graham, M. L., Mann, K. G., Spelsberg, T. C. and Riggs, B. L. (1988). Evidence of estrogen receptors in normal human osteoblast like cells. *Science*, **241**, 84–6.

68. Komm, B. S., Terpening, C. M., Benz, D. J., Graeme, K. A., Gallegos, A., Korc, M., Greene, G. L., O'Malley, B. W. and Haussler, M. R. (1988). Estrogen binding, receptor mRNA, and biologic response in osteoblast-like osteosarcoma cells. *Science*, **241**, 81–4.

69. Gray, T. K., Flynn, T. C., Gray, K. M. and Nabell, L. M. (1987). 17β-estradiol acts directly on the clonal osteoblast line UMR 106. *Proc. Natl. Acad. Sci. USA*, **84**. 6267–71.

70. Ernst, M., Schmid, C. and Froesch, E. R. (1988). Enhanced osteoblast proliferation and collagen gene expression by estradiol. *Proc. Natl. Acad. Sci. USA*, **85**, 2307–10.

71. Heaney, R. P. (1965). A unified theory of osteoporosis. *Am. J. Med.*, **39**, 877–80.

72. Jasani, C., Nordin, B. E. C., Smith, D. A. and Swanson, I. (1965). Spinal osteoporosis and the menopause. *Proc. Roy. Soc. Med.*, **58**, 441–4.

73. Rodan, G. A. and Martin, T. J. (1981). Role of osteoblasts in the hormonal control of bone resorption – a hypothesis. *Calcif. Tissue Int.*, **33**, 349–51.

74. Braidman, I. P., Anderson, D. C., Jones, C. J. P. and Weiss, J. B. (1983). Separation of two bone cell populations from fetal rat calvaria and a study of their responses to parathyroid hormone and calcitonin. *J. Endocrinol.*, **99**, 387–99.

75. McSheehy, P. M. J. and Chambers, T. J. (1986). Osteoblastic cells mediate osteoclastic responsiveness to parathyroid hormone. *Endocrinology*, **118**, 824–8.

76. Chambers, T. J., Anathanasou, N. A. and Fuller, K. (1984). Effect of parathyroid hormone and calcitonin on the cytoplasmic spreading of isolated osteoclasts. *J. Endrocrinol.*, **103**, 281–6.

77. Heath, H. and Sizemore, G. W. (1977). Plasma calcitonin in normal man. *J. Clin. Invest.*, **60**, 1135–40.

78. Parthemore, J. G. and Deftos, L. J. (1978). Calcitonin secretion in normal human subjects. *J. Clin. Endocrinol. Metab.*, **47**, 184–8.

79. Stevenson, J. C. (1985). Differential effects of aging and menopause on CT secretion. In Pecile, A. (ed.), *Calcitonin 1984: Chemistry, Physiology, Pharmacology and Clinical Aspects* (Amsterdam: Excerpta Medica), pp. 145–52.

80. Whitehead, M. I., Lane, G., Morsman, J., Myers, C. H. and Stevenson, J. C. (1984). Effect of castration on calcium regulating hormones. In Christiansen, C., Arnaud, C. D., Nordin, B. E. C., Parfitt, A. M., Peck, W. A. and Riggs, B. L. (eds), *Osteoporosis* (Glostrup, Denmark: Glostrup Hospital Clinical Chemistry Department), pp. 331–2.

81. Greenberg, C., Kukreja, S. C., Bowser, E. N., Hargis, G. K., Henderson, W. J. and Williams, G. A. (1986). Effects of estradiol and progesterone on calcitonin secretion. *Endocrinology*, **118**, 2594–8.

82. Williams, G. A., Kukreja, S. C., Bowser, E. N., Hargis, G. K., Greenberg,

C. P. and Henderson, W. J. (1986). Prolonged effect of estradiol on calcitonin secretion. *Bone and Mineral*, **1**, 415–20.

83. Morimoto, S., Tsuji, M., Okada, Y., Onishi, T. and Kumahara, Y. (1980). The effects of oestrogen on calcitonin secretion after calcium infusion in elderly female subjects. *Clin. Endocrinol.*, **13**, 135–43.

84. Stevenson, J. C., Abeyasekera, G., Hillyard, C. J., Phang, K. G., MacIntyre, I., Campbell, S., Townsend, P. T., Young, O. and Whitehead, M. I. (1981). Calcitonin and the calcium regulating hormones in postmenopausal women: effect of oestrogens. *Lancet*, **1**, 693–5.

85. Leggate, J., Farish, E., Fletcher, C. D., McIntosh, W., Hart, D. M. and Somerville, J. M. (1984). Calcitonin and postmenopausal osteoporosis. *Clin. Endocrinol.*, **20**, 85–92.

86. Selby, P. L., Peacock, M., Barkworth, S. A., Brown, W. B. and Taylor, G. A. (1985). Early effects of ethinyloestradiol and norethisterone treatment in postmenopausal women on bone resorption and calcium regulating hormones. *Clin. Sci.*, **69**, 265–71.

87. Torring, O., Bucht, E. and Sjoberg, H. E. (1985). Plasma calcitonin response to a calcium clamp. Influence of age and sex. *Horm. Metabol. Res.*, **17**, 536–9.

88. Torring, O., Bucht, E. and Sjoberg, H. E. (1987). The influence of sex steroid hormones on plasma calcitonin response to the calcium clamp in normal subjects. *J. Bone Mineral Res.*, **2**, 407–11.

89. McDermott, M., Kidd, G. S., Blue, P., Ghaed, V. and Hofeld, F. D. (1983). Reduced bone mineral content in totally thyroidectomised patients: possible effects of calcitonin deficiency. *J. Clin. Endocrinol. Metab,*, **56**, 936–9.

90. Hurley, D. L., Tiegs, R. D., Wahner, H. W. and Heath, H. (1987). Axial and appendicular bone mineral density in patients with long-term deficiency or excess of calcitonin. *N. Engl. J. Med.*, **317**, 537–41.

91. Milhaud, G., Benezech-Lefevre, M. and Moukhtar, M. S. (1978). Deficiency of calcitonin in age related osteoporosis. *Biomedicine*, **29**, 272–6.

92. Taggart, H. McA., Chesnut, C. H., Ivey, J. L., Baylink, D. J., Sisom, K., Huber, M. B. and Roos, B. A. (1982). Deficient calcitonin response to calcium stimulation in post menopausal osteoporosis? *Lancet*, **1**, 475–8.

93. Cundy, T., Heynen, G., Ackroyd, C., Kissin, M., Kibry, R. and Kanis, J. A. (1978). Plasma calcitonin in women. *Lancet*, **2**, 159 (letter).

94. Chesnut, C. H., Baylink, D. J., Sisom, K., Nelp, W. B. and Roos, B. A. (1980). Basal plasma immunoreactive calcitonin in postmenopausal osteoporosis. *Metabolism*, **29**, 559–62.

95. Tiegs, R. D., Body, J. J., Wahner, H. W., Barta, J., Riggs, B. L. and Heath, H. (1985). Calcitonin secretion in postmenopausal osteoporosis. *N. Engl. J. Med.*, **312**, 1097–1100.

96. Heaney, R. P., Recker, R. R. and Saville, P. D. (1978). Menopausal changes in calcium balance performance. *J. Lab. Clin. Med.*, **92**, 953–63.

97. Crilly, R. G., Francis, R. M. and Nordin, B. E. C. (1981). Steroid hormones, ageing and bone. *Clin. Endocrinol. Metab.*, **10**, 115–39.

98. Cannigia, A., Gennari, C., Borrella, G., Bencini, M., Cesari, L., Poggi, C. and Escobar, C. (1970). Intestinal absorption of calcium-47 after treatment with oral oestrogen-gestogens in senile osteoporosis. *Br. Med. J.*, **4**, 30–32.

99. Gallagher, J. C., Riggs, B. L. and DeLuca, H. F. (1980). Effect of estrogen

on calcium absorption and serum vitamin D metabolites in postmenopausal osteoporosis. *J. Clin. Endocrinol. Metab.*, **51**, 1359–64.

100. Civitelli, R., Agnusdei, D., Nardi, P., Zacchei, F., Avioli, L. V. and Gennari, C. (1988). Effects of one-year treatment with estrogens on bone mass, intestinal calcium absorption, and 25-hydroxyvitamin D-lα-hydroxylase reserve in postmenopausal osteoporosis. *Calcif. Tissue. Int.*, **42**, 77–86.

101. Tanaka, Y., Castillo, L. and DeLuca, H. F. (1976). Control of renal vitamin D hydroxylases in birds by sex hormones. *Proc. Natl. Acad Sci. USA*, **73**, 2701–5.

102. Baksi, S. N. and Kenny, A. D. (1977). Vitamin D_3 metabolism in immature Japanese quail: effects of ovarian hormones. *Endocrinology*, **101**, 1216–20.

103. Bouillon, R. and van Baelen, H. (1981). Transport of vitamin D. Significance of free and total concentrations of vitamin D metabolites. *Calcif. Tissue. Int.*, **33**, 451–3.

104. Bouillon, R., van Baelen, H. and de Moor, P. (1977). The measurement of the vitamin D binding protein in human serum. *J. Clin. Endocrinol. Metab.*, **45**, 225–31.

105. Selby, P. L. and Peacock, M. (1986). The effect of transdermal oestrogen on bone, calcium regulating hormones and liver in postmenopausal women. *Clin. Endocrinol.*, **25**, 543–7.

106. Chan, S. D. H., Chiu, D. K. H. and Atkins, D. (1984). Oophorectomy leads to a relative decrease in 1,25 dihydroxycholecalciferol receptors in rat jejunal villous cells. *Clin. Sci,*, **66**, 745–8.

107. Duursma, S. A., Bijlsma, J. W. J., van Paasen, H. C., van Buul-Offers, S. C. and Skottner-Lundin, A. (1984). Changes in serum somatomedin and growth hormone concentrations after three weeks' oestrogen substitution in postmenopausal women; a pilot study. *Acta Endocrinol.*, **106**, 527–31.

108. Feyen, J. H. M. and Raisz, L. G. (1987). Prostaglandin production by calvariae from sham operated and oophorectomised rats: effects of 17β-estradiol in vivo. *Endocrinology*, **121**, 819–21.

109. Gonzalez, D., Ghiringhelli, G. and Mautalen, C. (1986). Acute antiosteoclastic effect of salmon calcitonin in osteoporotic woman. *Calcif. Tissue Int.*, **38**, 71–5.

110. van Breukelen, F. J. M., Bijvoet, O. L. M., Frijlink, W. B., Sleeboom, H.P., Mulder, H. and van Oosterom, A. T. (1982). Efficacy of aminohydroxypropylidene bisphosphonate in hypercalcaemia. *Calcif. Tissue Int.*, **34**, 321–7.

111. Haussler, M. R., Donaldson, C.A., Allegretto, E. A., Marion, S. L., Mangelsdorf, D. J., Kelly, M. A. and Pike, J. W. (1984). New actions of 1,25-dihydroxyvitamin D_3: possible clues to the pathogenesis of osteoporosis. In Christiansen, C., Arnaud, C. D., Nordin, B. E. C., Parfitt, A. M., Peck, W. A. and Riggs, B. L. (eds), *Osteoporosis* (Glostrup, Denmark: Glostrup Hospital Clinical Chemistry Department), pp. 725–36.

112. Chambers, T. J. (1985). The pathobiology of the osteoclast. *J. Clin. Pathol.*, **38**, 241–52.

113. Souweine, G., Danel, L., Costa, O., Tubiana, N., Martin, P., Monier, J. C. and Saez, S. (1980). Effect of physiological concentrations of sex hormones on the formation of 'early' sheep red blood cell rosettes by human lymphocytes. Possible relations with the presence of sex-hormone-cytosol-receptors in lymphocytes. *Biomedicine*, **33**, 150–2.

114. Danel, L., Souweine, G., Monier, J. C. and Saez, S. (1983). Specific estrogen

binding sites in human lymphoid cells and thymic cells. *J. Steroid Biochem.*, **18,** 559–63.

115. Weusten, J. J. A. M., Blankenstein, M. A., Gmelig-Meyling, F. H. J., Schuurman, H. J., Kater, L. and Thijssen, J. H. H. (1986). Presence of oestrogen receptors in human blood mononuclear cells and thymocytes. *Acta Endocrinol.*, **112,** 409–14.
116. Fuller, K. and Chambers, T. J. (1987). Generation of osteoclasts in cultures of rabbit bone marrow and spleen cells. *J. Cell Physiol.*, **132,** 441–52.
117. Takahashi, N., Akatsu, T., Udasgawa, N., Sasaki, T., Yamaguchi, A., Moseley, J. M., Martin, T. J. and Suda, T. (1988). Osteoblastic cells are involved in osteoclast formation. *Endocrinology*, **123,** 2600–2.

5

CORTICOSTEROID OSTEOPOROSIS

D. M. REID

Ever since Cushing first described his syndrome in 1932 it has been recognized that supraphysiological levels of endogenous corticosteroids are associated with excessive bone loss. Cushing himself described spinal osteopenia in six of eight autopsied cases with adrenal hyperplasia[1] and radiological studies subsequently confirmed severe bone loss as part of the condition[2,3]. Indeed, endogenous Cushing's disease may well present with severe osteopenia, leading to multiple fractures[4]. The fractures occur at sites consisting principally of trabecular bone, especially the vertebrae and ribs, and have been estimated to occur in 20–67% of cases[2,3,5]. A recent review of 70 patients with the condition found a prevalence of osteoporosis of 50% and an incidence of spontaneous fractures of 19%[6]. It may be that peripheral fractures are relatively uncommon[6], and axial fractures are said to be more common in women[2,6], although this is not the experience of all[7].

The use of non-invasive bone mass and density assessment in endogenous Cushing's syndrome has confirmed the predilection for trabecular bone in the vertebrae but also in the femoral neck[8]. Other studies have failed to show cortical bone loss in the periphery[9,10] while showing substantial vertebral bone loss in purely trabecular bone in the vertebrae[10]. The loss of trabecular bone mass is certainly over 20% when quantified[8,10] and hence, despite there being only 20% of trabecular bone in the skeleton[11], it is of no surprise that five of seven patients reported have reduced total body calcium[12].

Almost immediately after the introduction of cortisone as a therapeutic agent in 1949[13], it became apparent that exogenous hyper-cortisonism was also associated with profound bone loss and most of the subsequent advances in our understanding of corticosteroid-induced osteoporosis have been made in the study of iatrogenic disease. Spontaneous fractures were first recorded in 1950 in two elderly patients receiving cortisone for the treatment of rheumatoid arthritis[14] and subsequently fractures were reported to occur in the vertebrae[15,16], ribs[16] and the pelvis[17,18].

A recent review of the published information on fracture rates in patients receiving corticosteroids arrived at a prevalence of 2–17%[19], but these figures were all based on studies carried out in the 1950s and 1960s using a variety of preparations including ACTH[20,21], corti-sone[22–24] and hydrocortisone[23]. Some of the more recent studies using semi-synthetic preparations, principally prednisone and prednisolone, will be discussed later in this chapter. Assessment of the prevalence of osteoporosis in patients treated with exogenous corticosteroids is fraught with difficulties because of the many variables which might influence the development of bone loss. Some of the variables which will be examined further in this review include the effects of daily dose of corticosteroids, the duration of therapy, the disease for which treatment is being prescribed and, more fundamentally, the site of bone loss and the age and sex of those at risk of osteoporosis. There are no case-control prospective studies reported to date investigating specifically fracture prevalence in those receiving corticosteroids. Despite this it is only the purest of the purists who would not accept the overwhelming evidence that corticosteroids are associated with the development of excess and early osteoporosis[25]. The remainder of this chapter will hopefully confirm the author's prejudice that the medication can be so implicated.

Influence of age and sex on the development of osteoporosis

Despite the use of non-invasive techniques of bone mass assessment, there remains controversy as to which group of patients are most at risk of developing osteoporosis. A recent consensus group felt that children were a group who were particularly at risk[26], perhaps especially girls[24], while others have suggested that premenopausal women[27], postmenopausal women[26,28,29] or even men[29,30] are most at risk, although in the latter report it may have been as a result of a higher corticosteroid dose[30].

Site of exogenous corticosteroid-induced bone loss

As expected, the bone loss associated with exogenous corticosteroids is said to be similar to that occurring with endogenous production and is mainly trabecular[31,32]. As referenced above the fractures occur principally at trabecular bone sites and the *in vivo* assessment of bone loss has confirmed this clinical observation. However initial studies of *in vivo* peripheral bone mass, using cortical thickness indices of the radial shaft, did show excess bone loss over and above that expected from the disease (rheumatoid arthritis) itself[33] and most studies using photon absorptiometry of the forearm, at sites consisting of both trabecular and cortical bone, have shown substantial reductions[34,35], although this is not the experience of all[36]. Studies where a proximal and distal forearm site has been measured have shown that bone loss is greater at the distal site[37-40], although in one study only in the first 12 weeks of therapy[41]. The contention that the distal site represented principally trabecular bone[40] was subsequently challenged[42] because of previous work showing that a site 2 cm proximal to the ulnar styloid contained only 24% of trabecular bone[43].

Use of dual-photon absorptiometry of the lumbar spine and other sites has demonstrated that bone loss is greatest in the lumbar spine, less in the proximal femur and least in the femoral shaft, the trend following the reduction in percentage of trabecular bone[44,45] and another study using single- and dual-photon absorptiometry showed minor reductions in bone density at both proximal and distal sites in the forearm with a marked reduction at the lumbar spine[46].

Despite the controversy as to the extent of cortical loss, the studies examining the total bone mass of corticosteroid-treated patients have invariably shown greater reductions in bone mass in corticosteroid-treated patients compared with disease controls[47-49], despite the skeleton consisting of 80% cortical bone[11]. However, a 6-month longitudinal study in patients with rheumatoid arthritis treated with low-dose corticosteroids failed to show any reduction in total body calcium[50], indicating either that the dose was too low to cause any damage or that the methodology was too imprecise.

There is a paucity of recent data on pure cortical bone in the hand, although a previous study did show a small reduction in cortical indices in a mixed group of corticosteroid-treated patients[51]. More recent studies have shown small doses of corticosteroids not to be associated with excess metacarpal[52] or hand bone mineral[53] loss in rheumatoid arthritis, and larger doses, as used in systemic lupus erythematosus, also seem to be free of such effects[54]. However, cortical indices have been found to be reduced in patients with asthma[55], although our data on hand bone mineral, measured by single-photon absorptiometry[56] show no reduction in this disorder[53].

In a single prospective longitudinal study measurements of pure trabecular bone in the distal tibia and 80% cortical bone at the radius showed dramatic bone loss at the trabecular site but an insignificant loss at the cortical site[57]. Recently Japanese workers have shown dramatic reductions in pure trabecular bone in the lumbar spine, as measured by QCT[58].

In summary, there is a great deal of evidence to support the contention that trabecular bone is affected adversely to a much greater extent than cortical bone by corticosteroid therapy, and this leads to increased fractures at bone sites with a high trabecular content. Cortical bone, however, seems to be much less affected, if at all, and perhaps accordingly there is little evidence that cortical fractures are increased in frequency in those on long-term corticosteroids. However, recent data in rats showing reduction in cortical bone strength after 90 days glucocorticoid therapy[59] may suggest caution in asserting that there is no increased risk of cortical fractures in humans.

PATHOPHYSIOLOGY OF GLUCOCORTICOID-INDUCED BONE LOSS

Although there has been an explosion of information on the possible aetiopathogenesis of corticosteroid-induced osteoporosis in the past 30 years, there are still many points of dispute in the literature. Both direct and indirect effects on bone remodelling are recognized, and will be highlighted in the next few pages. The principal pharmacological effects, may well be summarized by the statement that

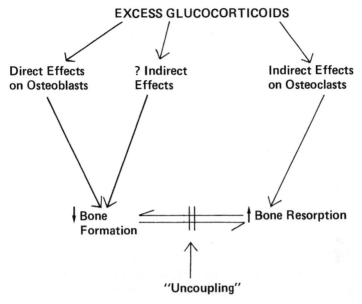

FIGURE 5.1   Summary of possible mechanisms of adverse effects of corticosteroids on bone metabolism

corticosteroids produce an indirect enhancement of resorption and a direct inhibition of formation, a situation likely to lead to a profound negative bone balance[60]. The possible mechanisms of the adverse effects are summarized in Figure 5.1. Much of the preliminary evidence for these effects has been derived from pathological studies of patients both with endogenous, and exogenous, Cushing's syndrome.

Bone microhistomorphometry – corticosteroid effects

Histological studies to date all show profound negative bone balance with resorption outstripping formation. Most authors have found evidence of increased bone resorption either by finding an increase in osteoclast number[51,61,62] or increased resorption surfaces[51,62–65], although neither definitively proves a dynamic increase in resorption rate[66]. Decreased osteoid thickness[67], decreased formation surfaces[63,68], decreased mineral apposition rates[62,64,65] and most importantly decreased mean wall thickness of trabecular packets[65,69], all give convincing evidence for a decrease in formation rate. Hence, bone histomorphometry has led investigators to search for reasons for the putative increase in bone resorption and the more definite decrease in bone formation. If both increased bone resorption and decreased bone formation coexist normal physiological coupling linking resorption to formation rate must be suppressed[32,66,70], and the dual effect on bone metabolism will lead to a profound reduction in bone mass, a situation which can be recognized histomorphometrically by reduced trabecular bone volume[35,66].

Bone resorption effects

As stated above, glucocorticoids clearly have the capacity to promote osteoclast accumulation in man[51,61,62]. The question remains as to whether this could be due to a direct stimulant effect of the hormones/drugs on bone resorption or whether it is an entirely secondary phenomenon. As osteoclasts are thought to be members of the monocyte–macrophage family[71], Teitelbaum and colleagues have developed assays based upon the use of pure populations of rat peritoneal macrophages as models of bone resorption[72]. Using this assay system they have shown that cortisol in physiological concentrations stimulates macrophage-mediated bone resorption[73], but such a finding is in direct contrast to the data from organ culture systems where high levels of corticosteroids inhibit bone resorption stimulated by several promoting agents[74–76]. This paradox may be explained by an inhibition of osteoclast differentiation by glucocorticoids[77] and *in vivo* the balance of evidence is in favour of an indirectly mediated stimulation of bone resorption[60].

Assuming an indirect effect, what are the possible explanations? There are many, and these are summarized in Figure 5.2. Calcium malabsorption clearly occurs with high-dose corticosteroids both in rats[78] and in man[79]. However, perhaps the effect is dose-dependent as in one study only daily doses of 15–100 mg were associated with calcium malabsorption, while lower daily doses (8–10 mg) or higher alternate-day doses (30–100 mg) were not[80]. Alternatively it may occur only in those who subsequently develop spinal osteoporosis, perhaps associated with reduced levels of 1,25-dihydroxyvitamin D[81].

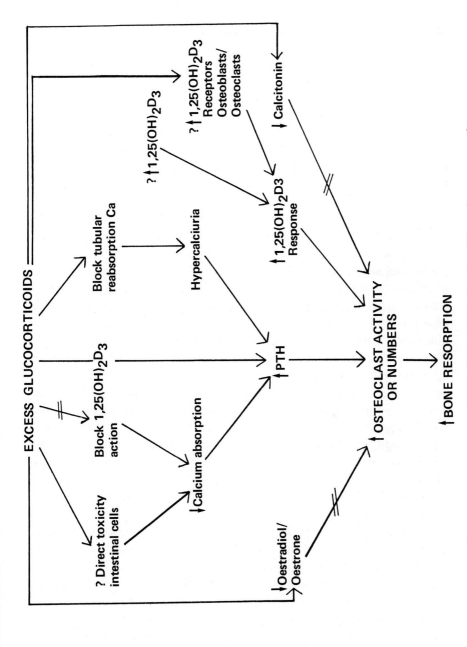

FIGURE 5.2   Possible effects of corticosteroids on bone resorption

Effects on vitamin D and its actions

The role of vitamin D metabolism in corticosteroid-induced osteoporosis is contentious. Because 1,25-dihydroxyvitamin D [1,25(OH)$_2$D$_3$] is the major regulator of intestinal calcium absorption, reduced production was considered to be a possible mechanism of calcium malabsorption[82]. Surprisingly 1,25(OH)$_2$D$_3$ has been shown to be *increased* with short-term corticosteroid therapy[79,83], and while reduced levels have been shown to occur in children with glomerulonephritis[84], perhaps related to reduced conversion of 25(OH)D$_3$ to the active metabolite in the kidney, most recent studies have shown normal values[85,86]. 25(OH)D$_3$ has also been found to be normal in endogenous Cushing's syndrome[12] and iatrogenic hypercortisonism[87], although with high-dose prednisolone it may be decreased[80,88].

On balance, therefore, it appears unlikely that disturbances in the levels of vitamin D metabolites or their production are responsible for calcium malabsorption, and indeed a single study has shown no relationship between circulating concentrations of vitamin D metabolites and calcium absorption in the presence of corticosteroids[79]. Accordingly the hypothesis of a decreased sensitivity of the gut wall to the effects of 1,25(OH)$_2$D$_3$ in the presence of corticosteroids has been raised[89]. Glucocorticoid receptors were first found in the small intestine of rats[90], and in this species glucocorticoids also cause calcium malabsorption while increasing sodium and glucose transport[78]. Active transport of other elements in man, including iron, have been found to be reduced[91] and, *in vitro*, cortisol inhibits calcium transport across gut cells[92]. Indirect evidence supporting the hypothesis comes from the observation of improvement in intestinal calcium transport in vitamin D-deficient rats[93] and in corticosteroid-treated patients[80] by the administration of 1,25(OH)$_2$D$_3$. Recently it has been shown that glucocorticoids competitively interfere with 1,25(OH)$_2$D$_3$ receptors in the intestines of rats[94] and dogs[95].

It remains possible that the effects of 1,25(OH)$_2$D$_3$ in the presence of glucocorticoids may not be at gut level, but may be due to a direct effect on osteoclasts, probably via an effect on osteoblasts and the coupling mechanism (see below). 1,25(OH)$_2$D$_3$ clearly induces bone resorption[96], although osteoclasts appear to lack vitamin D receptors[97]. Whether an up-regulation of vitamin D receptors in bone cells in the presence of corticosteroids could increase the resorbing effects of the drugs in humans remains to be proven[98].

Effects on parathyroid hormone (PTH)

Histological evidence for increased bone resorption suggests that glucocorticoids may induce a state of secondary hyperparathyroidism thought to result from a relative fall in serum calcium due to the reduction in intestinal calcium absorption[82]. Although corticosteroids do not cause frank hypocalcaemia, the tendency to reduced levels may be enhanced by hypercalciuria, which is certainly induced by dexamethasone[99] and by high-dose prednisolone[100]. In addition glucocorticoids can directly release PTH from rat parathyroid glands in organ culture[101] and this has also been demonstrated in man[102]. Immunoreactive PTH has been found to be slightly above normal in most[63,100,102–104], but not all studies[105]. Further evidence for the effects of PTH in inducing corticosteroid-induced bone resorption comes from studies in animals where parathyroidectomy completely abolishes the osteoclastic response[106].

As PTH receptors have not been described on osteoclasts, a communication system between PTH-activated osteoblasts and osteoclasts has been postulated[107]. Glucocorticoids seem to increase the sensitivity of osteoblasts to PTH[108] and hence bone resorption may be increased by enhancing the putative communication system between PTH-activated osteoblasts and osteoclasts[109].

Corticosteroid effects on other hormones and cytokines involved in bone resorption

The possible indirect effects of a reduction in the hormones which might protect against bone resorption have received little literature attention. However, it has been shown in a single study that immunoreactive calcitonin was reduced after the introduction of corticosteroids in seven patients treated for a variety of different disorders, while no change was noted in PTH or urinary cyclic AMP[110]. In addition, recent evidence has shown a reduced calcitonin response to calcium infusion in patients receiving 1 month of corticosteroid therapy[98] and an effect of the hormone is given some credence by the

111

observation that calcitonin retards some of the detrimental effects of corticosteroids on bone in rabbits[111].

The effect of sex steroids on bone resorption has recently been considered. Levels of oestrone, androstenedione and oestradiol have all been shown to be decreased in postmenopausal corticosteroid-treated patients compared to controls[112], although low androgen levels in postmenopausal women may have a negative effect on bone formation rather than a direct effect on bone resorption[113]. Recent evidence from cultures of pig granulosa cells has shown a direct effect on oestradiol secretion by several corticosteroids[114].

The possibility that corticosteroid effects on bone resorption might be mediated by the release of locally produced cytokines has recently received attention[115]. However, many of the local mediators of bone resorption such as interleukin-1[116], tumour necrosis factor[117] and bradykinin[118] have their secretion reduced or their effects inhibited by glucocorticoid action[115], and the complexity of these changes at the local bone level is yet to be fully investigated.

The full effects of corticosteroids on bone resorption remain to be fully elucidated. Much of the contradictory evidence presented from humans relates to the different doses of prednisolone or equivalent used, and the time of study in relation to the onset of therapy. *In vivo* effects of increased bone resorption have received scant attention and, for example, there is little information on the production of collagen breakdown products such as urinary hydroxyproline in patients under treatment. Where measured it has been shown to be increased with short-term relatively high-dose corticosteroid therapy[104,119], while in those established on moderate-dose therapy it is normal[120-122]. While effects on bone resorption could be dose-related, it remains possible that increased bone resorption is only present for a short time after the introduction of corticosteroids, and thereafter returns to a normal or even low level in parallel with bone formation.

Bone formation effects

Much of the recent histomorphometric data has shown evidence of a decrease in bone formation in patients receiving exogenous corticosteroids (see above). The possible reasons for this observation are

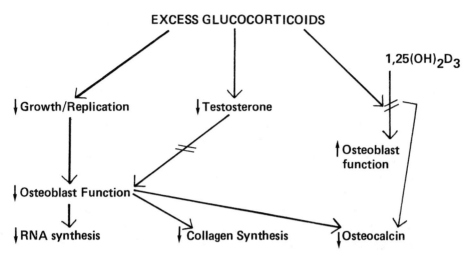

FIGURE 5.3   Major effects of corticosteroids on bone formation

summarized in Figure 5.3. Glucocorticoid receptors have been found in osteogenic sarcoma cells and in homogenated bone tissue[123–125], and in these *in vitro* situations glucocorticoids may have a direct inhibitory effect[107,126]. Some workers have suggested that the effect on osteoblasts is not on mature forms, but on their precursors[127], and that pro-staglandin synthesis inhibition may be responsible for some of this effect[128]. Whatever the mechanism, glucocorticoids appear to have a suppressive effect on protein and RNA synthesis on isolated bone cells *in vitro*[129,130], although in cultured calvariae there may be an early stimulant effect, followed by a later inhibitory effect after long-term exposure[126,127].

Whether this work, carried out principally on fetal rat calvariae or rat osteogenic sarcoma cell lines, can appropriately be applied to the human situation is debatable. However, there is indirect evidence from human osteoblastic cell lines to support the inhibitory effects of glucocorticoids on the cells. The evidence is based on the production by osteoblasts of the low molecular weight protein, osteocalcin (also known as bone Gla protein or BGP)[131]. The synthesis of this protein, which reflects osteoblastic activity, is inhibited by glucocorticoids *in vitro*[132] and interestingly also in corticosteroid-treated patients *in vivo*[133–135], perhaps especially women[136]. The fall in osteocalcin may occur within 1 week of the onset of therapy[137], but appears to be persistent and may indicate continuing reduction in bone formation.

The inhibitory effects on osteoblasts of glucocorticoids could be influenced by $1,25(OH)_2D_3$. Receptors for this hormone have been found on osteoblasts of rats[138] and mice[139], among other species. Recent work suggests that glucocorticoids can up-regulate the receptors on rat osteoblasts[138], while down-regulating them on mice osteoblasts[139]. The effects of corticosteroids on vitamin D receptors on human osteoblasts is unclear[109], but $1,25(OH)_2D_3$ can stimulate alkaline phosphatase production and collagen synthesis[140], while inhibiting cell proliferation[140]. If glucocorticoids were responsible for down-regulation of vitamin D receptors on human osteoblasts, the effects of $1,25(OH)_2D_3$ would be reduced, and could therefore be responsible for reduced bone matrix formation. However, if this were the case $1,25(OH)_2D_3$-induced bone resorption[96], which may result from a primary action on osteoblasts to induce a coupling factor capable of stimulating osteoclastic bone resorption[141], would also be reduced. Nevertheless, simultaneous administration of $1,25(OH)_2D_3$ to rats overcomes the glucocorticoid-induced suppression of osteocalcin production[142].

All the evidence reported so far suggests a direct effect of glucocorticoids on osteoblasts as the final common pathway of inhibition of bone formation. However, the possibility of an indirect effect on sex steroids should not be overlooked. Exogenous glucocorticoids acutely reduce the testosterone levels in men[143] and levels are also reduced in female patients established on therapy[112,113]. While ACTH has been shown to increase testosterone levels in women, suggesting that suppression of ACTH production is responsible[112], more recent work has suggested that the reduced testosterone levels in men are due to reduced secretion of gonadotrophin releasing hormone[143]. The stimulus to attempt therapy of corticosteroid-induced osteoporosis with anabolic steroids is obvious.

The observations that calmodulin, a multifunctional calcium-dependent modulating protein, is elevated in steroid-treated rabbit bone[144] and that plasma selenium is reduced in corticosteroid-treated patients with rheumatoid arthritis[145], remain to be fully elucidated as far as bone formation and resorption are concerned.

On balance the evidence from the studies quoted above would suggest that the dramatic effects of exogenous corticosteroids on bone mass are due to an unusual combination of increased bone resorption and decreased bone formation occurring at one and the same time. Such a conclusion would obviously entail a breakdown in the normal mechanism 'coupling' the two sides of the bone metabolism equation. This aspect of corticosteroid effects must remain speculative, and will only be resolved when the cytokine which drives the coupling mechanism has been clearly isolated and identified. Much of the contradictory evidence from studies in humans must relate to factors of clinical importance, such as the dose and duration of corticosteroid therapy and the disease for which the drugs are being prescribed. The effects of dose of glucocorticoids, in particular, may make the interpretation of studies involving isolated bone cells *in vitro*, bone culture techniques and even studies involving living animals difficult to interpret in the human context. Nevertheless it remains possible from the evidence described above that corticosteroids have their main effect in inducing rapid bone turnover (by increased bone resorption) early in the course of therapy, when the dose used may be fairly high in any case, and then have a later effect on inhibiting bone turnover (by reduced bone formation *and* reduced bone resorption). Such a hypothesis, if true, would have profound effects on the choice of corticosteroid regimes of therapy, and particularly in developing preventative measures and treatment regimes for established osteoporosis.

CLINICAL FEATURES OF CORTICOSTEROID INDUCED OSTEOPOROSIS

Fractures

Exogenous corticosteroids are widely used in many branches of clinical medicine, but because of their particular use in the management of rheumatic and pulmonary disease, much of the clinical research has been carried out within these two disciplines. The presentation of corticosteroid-induced osteoporosis is usually with a fracture. From the evidence already presented it is obvious that the drugs have their most profound effect on trabecular bone. It is not surprising, therefore, that an increased incidence of fractures was first reported in the vertebral bodies in patients with rheumatic diseases[14–17,24,147], but interestingly it was not until 1983 that the clinically well-recognized rib fractures occurring in patients with asthma were recognized[40]. It is assumed that these occur because of persistent coughing[40], although they do also occur in patients with rheumatoid arthritis[16].

TABLE 5.1 Fracture incidence in patients treated with exogenous glucocorticoids

Reference	Disease	No.	Prevalence (%)	Sites	Dose (mg/day)	Duration of therapy (years)
Adinoff and Hollister[40]	Asthma	128	11	ribs/vert.	30*	8*
Verstraeten and Dequeker[28]	RA	28	16.3	vert./fem.n.	8.9	4.7
Dykman et al.[149]	RA/SLE	93	18	vert.	15.6	4.0
Badley and Ansell[24]	JCA	63	15	vert./others	25–†100	1.4–2.7
Hahn et al.[147]	RA	103	17.5	vert.	17.5	4.6
Luengo et al.[148]	Asthma	35	20	vert.	8.0	8.5

*Mean dose and duration of steroids at time of fracture
†Daily dose of cortisone
Abbreviations
No.   = Number included in study
Dose   = Daily dose of prednisolone or equivalent
RA   = Rheumatoid arthritis
SLE   = Systemic lupus erythematosus
JCA   = Juvenile chronic arthritis
Vert.   = Vertebral bodies
Fem.n. = Femoral neck

The incidence of fractures has not been studied systematically or prospectively, but a summary of the retrospective studies (Table 5.1) shows a remarkable percentage similarity ranging from 11% to 20%, despite the greatly differing numbers of patients studied and the different doses and duration of corticosteroids used. Spontaneous fractures occur at other sites including the femur[16], pelvis[17,18] and humerus[149]. Whether fractures at these extravertebral sites are increased in prevalence due to corticosteroid therapy is far from clear. Of particular concern would be an increase in the risk of femoral neck fractures, and corticosteroid therapy has been suggested to be an independent risk factor in postmenopausal women[150]. In a study examining possible risk factors for the development of fracture of the neck of femur, corticosteroids could not be definitely identified as an independent risk factor, but the fractures were shown to occur at an earlier age[151]. In a retrospective study in Edinburgh, my colleagues and I were unable to show an increased prevalence of rheumatoid arthritis in patients with hip fractures despite the use of corticosteroids in over 20% of the fracture population[152].

Vertebral and rib fractures, therefore, are increased in frequency with corticosteroid therapy, but the data on other fractures are inconclusive. As it has been demonstrated that the mean reduction in total bone mass in those with postmenopausal vertebral fractures is 16–20%[153–155], it is obvious that substantial bone loss predates fractures. There have been no published attempts to screen at-risk populations to detect those individuals who may be developing glucocorticoid-induced osteoporosis. Although radiographs are notoriously unreliable in detecting bone loss, it being frequently stated that 30% of bone mass must be lost before it becomes radiologically obvious[156,157], it would seem reasonable to screen patients who are to be commenced on corticosteroids for pre-existing vertebral osteoporosis. Any more intensive screening of corticosteroid-treated patients would have to use one of the newer *in vivo* methods of bone mass assessment. Diagnosis of bone loss after therapy has been commenced could be achieved by screening, but in practice it is usually not considered until a fracture occurs, when the effect of the drug may be difficult to differentiate from age- or menopause-associated bone loss. Perhaps insufficient note has been taken of the suggestion that the vertebral radiological changes associated with therapy are specific and different from idiopathic osteoporosis in that, instead of losing horizontal trabeculae with consequent prominence of vertical trabeculae, all the trabeculae (horizontal and vertical) are said to become uniformly narrowed[158].

Degree of bone loss

The extent of bone loss associated with corticosteroids can only be surmised from fracture data, but many studies have examined the problem using *in vivo* bone mass assessment techniques. The data from those studies, giving details of the disease treated and the dose and duration of therapy, are summarized in Table 5.2. The loss of bone mass varies between 4.0% and 35.2%, depending on the site of bone mass examined, the dose and duration of corticosteroids used and the disease for which the medication has been prescribed. Again most of the data has been derived from patients with rheumatic and pulmonary diseases. Some of the discrepancies occurring in Table 5.2 are based on the profound local bone loss which occurs as a feature of rheumatoid arthritis[49,159]. In studies examining patients with rheumatoid arthritis only, the smallest reduction in peripheral bone, where bone mass has been assessed by single-photon absorptiometry (SPA) of the forearm, is 14% at a proximal site and 28.5% at a distal site[39]. However, in asthma, bone mass at the proximal site has been reported as normal, while at the distal site it is reduced by only 15%[40]. In rheumatoid arthritis two studies failed to show a significant reduction in spine bone mineral content[28,160], while another showed only a small reduction in female patients[161].

Disease specificity of bone loss

It was almost certainly the type of discrepancy described above, associated with the use of SPA of the forearm, that led Mueller to conclude that corticosteroid-induced bone loss was greater in patients receiving equal doses of the drugs for rheumatoid arthritis (RA) than it was those receiving therapy for asthma[162]. Hahn and colleagues

---

Abbreviations for Table 5.2

RA	= Rheumatoid arthritis
SLE	= Systemic lupus erythematosus
Red.	= Mean percentage reduction compared with controls
Dose	= Daily dose of prednisolone or equivalent
CTD	= Connective tissue disease
SPA	= Single-photon absorptiometry (P = proximal forearm; D = distal forearm)
Trab.Vol.	= Trabecular volume at the iliac crest
TBCa	= Total-body calcium
TBBM	= Total-body bone mineral by DPA
DPA	= Dual-photon absorptiometry (S = lumbar spine; FN = femoral neck; FS = femoral shaft)
QCT.T	= Quantitative computed tomography at the tibia

TABLE 5.2 Degree of bone loss in corticosteroid treated patients

Reference	Disease	No.	Red. (%)	Method	Dose (mg/day)	Duration of therapy (years)
Hahn[31]	RA/others	33	17.4 39.3	SPA.P SPA.D	14.7	9.4
Chesney et al.[84]	Renal	25	16.7	SPA	>2.5	4.8
Nordin et al.[121]	?	32	35.2	Trab. Vol.	5–20	?
Gluck et al.[38]	RA/SLE/CTD	25	16.3 17.1	SPA.P SPA.D	12.8	7.8
Reid et al.[48]	RA	32	15.5,F 11.5,M	TBCa	6.3 6.1	6.6 2.7
Als et al.[49]	RA	13	26 32	TBBM SPA.D	2.5–10	?
Ruegsegger et al.[57]	Asthma	20	13	QCT.T	12.5	>1
Adinoff and Hollister[40]	Asthma	19	1 15	SPA.P SPA.D	?	>1
Als et al.[122]	RA	24	27	SPA.D	2.5–10	6.1
Schadt and Bohr[45]	Various	30	19.5 9.0 5.7	DPA.S DPA.FN DPA.FS	8.5	7.3
Dykman et al.[149]	Various	23	14.0 28.5	SPA.P SPA.D	11.8	5.9
Sambrook et al.[159]	RA	44	9.6 12.2	DPA.S DPA.FN	8.0	7.5
Verstraeten and Dequeker[28]	RA	28	4.0	DPA.S	8.9	5.6
Reid et al.[164]	Asthma	22	13.6	TBCa	6.8	12.5
Luengo et al.[148]	Asthma	35	14	DPA.S	8.0	8.5

showed very similar findings comparing patients with RA and those with other diseases, although the authors drew no conclusions from the observation[37]. In our studies in Edinburgh a similar conclusion was reached from preliminary analysis of total bone mass studies using total body calcium (TBCa), i.e. that patients with RA were more susceptible to the adverse effects of corticosteroids on bone than patients with asthma or polymyalgia rheumatica[163]. Full analysis of the data suggested that our preliminary assessment had been incorrect and, allowing for the effects of RA on bone mass in general, there was no difference between the values of TBCa in patients with RA or asthma[164]. Interestingly the total bone mass of a small group of patients with polymyalgia rheumatica (PMR) remained significantly higher than either of the other two diseases studied. It was felt that this finding might be artefactual because of the elderly population and the very substantial 1.5% per annum menopausal correction which was used in the analysis[164]. Subsequently other small studies of patients with PMR have shown small reductions in lumbar spine bone density in those receiving therapy for over 3 years[165], but no reduction in bone density at the os calcis[166]. However, if there is a tendency for patients with PMR to lose less bone it does not appear to be due to a pharmacokinetic effect of prednisolone therapy[167].

A study investigating histomorphometric effects in the iliac crest showed no statistical difference in any of the derived parameters between patients with respiratory disease and those with connective tissue disorders[69].

In conclusion it seems likely that bone loss occurs with the use of corticosteroids in every disease, provided that the drugs are used for a long enough period of time and in a big enough dose.

Duration of treatment and bone loss

It is apparent that bone loss associated with the use of corticosteroids starts almost immediately the drugs are introduced. Fractures have been reported to occur as little as 1 month after the onset of treatment[168]. Animal studies have given support to this rapid bone loss, although in rabbit bone cells the loss becomes apparent only after 60 days of therapy, and tails off after 110 days[106]. Histological studies confirmed an initial increase in osteoclasts and resorption surfaces with a subsequent fall-off to a steady state which took 6–8 weeks in the rabbit, 2–3 months in the dog and approximately 4 months in the human[169]. Thus the increase in bone resorption occurring with corticosteroids may appear early in the course of therapy and may be a fairly transient event. Certainly some of the early histological studies of patients with established endogenous Cushing's syndrome of several years duration showed very little cellular activity[170].

The evidence for such effects in humans *in vivo* is limited and somewhat contradictory. Rapid effects have been shown to occur with an increase in hydroxyproline excretion, a decrease in intestinal calcium absorption and an increase in urinary calcium in the first 30 days of therapy[35]. Whether the lack of similar findings in some of the studies previously referenced can be laid at the door of a longer duration of corticosteroid therapy when bone resorption has already returned to more normal levels remains speculative.

Assessment of bone mass *in vivo* has given some support to the hypothesis of a rapid decline in bone mass in the first few months of therapy and a slower rate of loss thereafter. A 6-month longitudinal study showed a significant loss of bone from the distal forearm measured by SPA after 3 months of therapy, but no further loss in the following 3 months[171]. Initial studies published by my colleagues and me showed a significant correlation between the daily dose of prednisolone and the degree of bone loss in patients with RA receiving an unchanging daily dose[48]. No such correlations were shown with the duration of therapy or the total dose of prednisolone received. This suggested to us that the adverse effects of corticosteroids were occurring principally early in therapy, perhaps in the first year[48]. A subsequent longitudinal study investigating largely the same group of patients showed no continuing bone loss in those persisting with prednisolone therapy[172], these findings being similar to a previous investigation of TBCa in five patients who had diseases other than RA[173]. However, the cumulative dose has been suggested to be the most important factor in inducing fractures[149], and several other groups have suggested that the degree of bone loss correlates with the duration of therapy[31,35,37,174,175] although in the latter study it was suggested that the high-dose early phase of therapy may be the most important[175]. Longitudinal data from histomorphometric studies have shown dramatic losses of trabecular bone volume after 7 months of therapy which could not be sustained[176], and a longer study by the same group lasting over 12 months has confirmed that the initial rate of bone loss does not continue[177]. Studies of spinal bone mineral over 4 years in four asthmatic patients commencing corticosteroids have confirmed the rapid loss of bone in the first year of treatment, with only age-associated loss thereafter[98].

In summary there is increasing evidence that the most rapid period of bone loss after the introduction of corticosteroids is within the first few months of therapy, with a much more gradual loss, perhaps only that associated with ageing, thereafter. It is tempting to assume that the rapid phase of bone loss is due to an early effect of the drugs in increasing bone resorption while the effect on suppression of bone formation may be longer-lasting.

Dosage of glucocorticoids inducing bone loss

If it is correct that the major histochemical and catabolic effects of corticosteroids are occurring early in the course of therapy, then the daily dose of corticosteroids may well be the most important factor in determining whether osteoporosis supervenes. Is there a safe dose?

Malabsorption of calcium appears to occur only with higher doses of prednisolone or equivalent, 15–20 mg/day[80,89] being associated with decreased calcium absorption but 8–10 mg/day having no such effect[80]. The effects of daily dose and duration of therapy on the degree of bone loss *in vivo*, where reported and significant, are shown in Table 5.2. Studies where some of the patients were taking as little as 2.5 mg of prednisolone/day, have shown significant group reductions in bone mass[27,49,84]. However the lowest mean dose inducing significant bone loss is 6.3 mg/day[48], although we have shown that patients with RA taking a mean dose of 5 mg/day have decreased TBCa compared to that predicted from the activity and duration of their disease[178].

Radiological osteoporosis has been reported to be in excess of expected in RA patients taking only 5 mg/day, but the difference compared with RA patients not receiving corticosteroids was not significant[179]. Fractures have been noted in patients taking 5 mg[180] and 7.5 mg/day[16].

There is little evidence that calcium malabsorption is associated with very low dose corticosteroids, and certainly there appears to be no effect of 5 mg of prednisolone/day on vitamin D metabolism when studied prospectively[181]. Little is published on other aspects of bone resorption, but on the bone formation side of the equation there is evidence suggesting doses as low as 5–10 mg of prednisolone/day can be associated with a decreased osteoblastic effect[182].

In summary there is increasing evidence that even low doses of oral corticosteroids (< 10 mg/day) can be associated with reduced bone mass in susceptible patients, although perhaps the mechanism of action, particularly effects on bone resorption, are not so clearly defined as in patients on 15–20 mg/day or more. It certainly appears that there is, not unexpectedly, a dose effect with bone loss being significantly greater in patients with RA receiving 5.1–10 mg of prednisolone/day compared with those receiving < 5 mg/day in a cross-sectional study[178] and in a longitudinal study, in patients with asthma, the rate of loss over 12 months was increased in those taking higher doses of corticosteroids[57].

PREVENTION OF CORTICOSTEROID-INDUCED OSTEOPOROSIS

The possible methods of preventing the adverse effects of corticosteroids on bone are listed in Table 5.3. Obviously unnecessary corticosteroid prescription should be avoided, the lowest possible dose used and the medication discontinued as soon as possible[183], but an additional therapeutic medication or alternative methods of prescribing corticosteroids to prevent or reduce osteoporosis, while maintaining the beneficial anti-inflammatory effect, would be very useful.

Alternative methods of corticosteroid administration

Early retrospective studies suggested that ACTH was associated with very little osteoporosis[184] and few fractures[185]. However, it soon became clear that fractures did occur in those receiving long-term ACTH[20,21]. The suggestion that some of the adverse effects of corticosteroids could be due to a reduction in testosterone[112,113,143], an

TABLE 5.3 Possible preventive measures for corticosteroid-induced osteoporosis

A:	Alternative delivery methods	ACTH
		Intravenous methylprednisolone
		Inhaled corticosteroids
		Alternate-day therapy
B:	Add-on therapy	Calcium
		Sodium fluoride
		Oestrogens
		Vitamin D and metabolites
		Bisphosphonates
C:	Alternative steroids	Deflazacort

effect reversed by ACTH stimulation[112], could give some theoretical support for the use of ACTH as an alternative medication. There may be scope for examining this suggestion further using *in vivo* bone mass assessment.

Intravenous methylprednisolone in large doses has become popular intermittent therapy in the treatment of patients with rheumatic diseases, and in the field of transplant surgery. It is not likely that it will supplant daily oral corticosteroids, but investigators have given some thought as to whether it interferes with bone metabolism. Although there were transient increases in serum calcium, PTH and $1,25(OH)_2D_3$ in one study, the values of urinary hydroxyproline decreased[186]. A more recent study by the same authors confirmed most of the original findings, but suggested that the acute effect on serum calcium was reversed after 24 hours with increased urinary calcium excretion and a secondary rise in PTH[187]. Another study showed a decrease in serum calcium 1 week after therapy, with preservation of forearm bone mineral content at 4 and 8 months after treatment[188], a finding supported by results of cortical indices in the hand in a 6-month study of repeated pulses of methylprednisolone[189]. It seems unlikely that infrequent pulses of intravenous corticosteroids, even in large doses, will have any lasting adverse effect on bone metabolism.

The effects of inhaled corticosteroids used in the treatment of asthma have received little attention in the literature. My colleagues and I have shown total-body calcium to be reduced by a mean of 8.8% in patients with asthma receiving such therapy as their only continuous corticosteroid therapy, although many of the patients had also received booster courses of oral corticosteroids[164]. The trend for increasing use of high-dose corticosteroid inhalers[190] in the management of asthma suggests that users should be vigilant for the development of osteoporosis.

The use of alternate-day corticosteroid therapy to minimize the adverse effects of glucocorticoids on the hypothalamic–pituitary–adrenal axis has been recognized for many years, although there is debate as to whether such therapy reduces other adverse effects[191]. As far as the effects on bone are concerned, there is evidence that the inhibition of bone growth in children known to occur with daily therapy is less with alternate-day treatment[192], although this was not the case in children treated for glomerular disease[84]. In adults, the use of alternate-day regimes of corticosteroid therapy has been associated with trabecular bone loss in the tibia[57] and a similar degree of bone loss at the distal forearm site to that of patients taking daily corticosteroids, despite a slightly greater daily dose equivalent in the latter group[38]. Bone density was also shown to be reduced compared to disease controls in children receiving corticosteroids for renal disease[84].

Concomitant drug administration to prevent osteoporosis

Several agents have been suggested to have such an effect. In our own studies, asthmatic patients who had received oral calcium supplements along with corticosteroids had a slightly greater total bone mass than patients who had not received calcium supplements, despite the former group having taken prednisolone in a higher daily dose for a longer period of time[164]. Previous work has suggested that forearm bone mineral loss in patients established on corticosteroids is less with additional calcium prescription[193], and that some indices of bone resorption are reduced[194].

Sodium fluoride could be considered to be a preventive or a therapeutic agent, depending on whether it is prescribed at the onset of therapy or after patients are established on treatment and may have already developed bone loss. In mice sodium fluoride given orally and concomitantly with prednisolone failed to prevent the development of

125

osteoporosis[195], and similar data has been derived from a short-term study in humans[41,171].

Although it is suggested that postmenopausal women who require corticosteroids should also receive oestrogen replacement therapy if appropriate[29], such an approach does not prevent osteoporosis in mice[196], and might only prevent menopausal bone loss in women.

The role of vitamin D metabolites in the *prevention* of corticosteroid-induced osteoporosis has received little attention in humans, although they have been studied as a treatment of established disease (see below) and were included in small doses in the preventive therapeutic studies with fluoride[41,171]. Studies in animals with $1,25(OH)_2D_3$ as a preventive measure have produced conflicting results with benefit, especially on calcium absorption in rats[197,198], but no benefit on bone density in rabbits.

As bone resorption is a feature of early corticosteroid-induced osteoporosis, at least, it would seem reasonable to attempt to block osteoclastic bone resorption with bisphosphonate therapy. This approach has been found to be useful in rabbits treated with ethane diphosphonate[200], but the use of these agents as a preventive measure in those not previously receiving corticosteroids has yet to be tried in humans.

Alternative corticosteroids

The development of a corticosteroid with similar anti-inflammatory properties to prednisolone but with a decreased effect on bone would be advantageous. The discovery of an oxaziline derivative of prednisolone with these apparent effects (deflazacort) should be widely appreciated[201], although it is not yet widely available. This agent has been found to have clinical efficacy similar to prednisone in patients with rheumatoid arthritis and systemic lupus erythematosus[202], perhaps at a dose ratio of 6:5 mg[203]. *In vitro* it has a calcium-sparing effect on rat calvaria[204], and although it had no effect in preventing calcium malabsorption in human volunteers, it did have a reduced effect on the development of increased urinary calcium compared to prednisone[119]. In longitudinal studies in patients it has been shown to be associated with reduced bone loss at the iliac crest[176] and at the lumbar spine[205,206]. The mechanism of this apparent bone-sparing effect without decreasing anti-inflammatory efficacy has not been elucidated, and is difficult to understand in the present state of our knowledge of the glucocorticoid receptor.

More studies are required to investigate the effects of deflazacort, as well as further investigation of the role of vitamin D, calcitonin and bisphosphonates in the prevention of bone loss.

TREATMENT OF ESTABLISHED BONE DISEASE

The therapeutic modalities which have been tried or suggested in the treatment of osteoporosis in patients established on corticosteroids are shown in Table 5.4. Some of these treatments have been reported as measures to prevent osteoporosis, and not all the patients included

TABLE 5.4   Possible treatment regimes for corticosteroid-induced osteoporosis

Drugs to decrease bone resorption	Vitamin D and metabolites Calcitonin Biphosphonates
Drugs to increase bone formation	Sodium fluoride Anabolic steroids

in the studies outlined in the following paragraphs had suffered an osteoporotic fracture. Nevertheless, it seems illogical to consider drugs given to patients established on long-term corticosteroids as preventive therapy when the patients will almost certainly already have lost bone due to the initial glucocorticoid treatment.

If corticosteroids can be withdrawn there might be an improvement in the bone disease. This has certainly been shown to occur in endogenous Cushing's syndrome with an increase in bone mineral density at several sites, a decrease in urinary hydroxyproline and an increase in serum osteocalcin in one study[8], and a decrease in PTH and $1,25(OH)_2D_3$ in another[207]. Histological studies in endogenous[64,65], and exogenous[31] Cushing's syndrome reveal a dramatic increase in osteoblastic activity after therapy for the former or cessation of the latter.

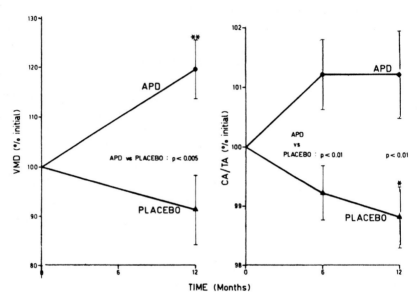

FIGURE 5.4   Vertebral mineral density (VMD) and metacarpal cortical area (expressed as a ratio to total area, CA/TA) as percentage of initial values in glucocorticoid-treated patients receiving either oral APD or placebo (from ref. 211, reproduced by kind permission of the authors and *The Lancet*)

Drugs to decrease bone resorption

The confusing effects of exogenous glucocorticoids on vitamin D metabolites have been discussed above. The finding of calcium malabsorption in most studies stimulated the idea of attempting to control or reverse the bone loss with vitamin D supplements. Initial studies showed the value of 25OH vitamin D, with calcium supplements, in increasing forearm bone mass and decreasing osteoclast number[62]. The improvement stimulated studies with the more active metabolite of the vitamin, $1,25(OH)_2D_3$. A dose of $2\,\mu g$ of $1\alpha\text{-}(OH)D_3$, used over

6 months in a double-blind study, raised intestinal calcium absorption and urinary calcium excretion, reduced PTH and urinary hydroxyproline, and decreased active bone resorption without apparently interfering with osteoblast function[120]. A more recent study of 1 μg of the same preparation of vitamin D showed an increase in urinary calcium with no significant change in forearm or spinal bone mineral content[208]. Use of the preparation $1,25(OH)_2D_3$ in a mean dose of 0.4 μg/day increased calcium absorption, decreased PTH and decreased osteoclast number, but it also decreased some parameters of osteoblastic activity, suggesting that the preparation should not be used therapeutically[39]. In any case, care should be exercised as calcium and vitamin D preparations can cause considerable hypercalcaemia[209].

Salmon calcitonin given subcutaneously in a dose of 100 IU on alternate days for 6 months significantly improved forearm bone mineral content compared with disease controls in a recent study[210], and with the development of nasal calcitonin this mode of therapy requires further study.

Bisphosphonates have been mentioned as possible preventive therapy. Recent work has suggested that (3-amino-1-hydroxypropylidene)-1,1-bisphosphonate (APD) with calcium supplements is useful in reversing the trend to bone loss with an increase in metacarpal cortical area (CA/TA) and vertebral mineral density (VMD) compared with disease controls receiving only calcium (Figure 5.4)[211]. This interesting study requires corroboration.

Drugs to increase bone formation

As there is reproducible suppression of bone formation in patients receiving corticosteroids, it is logical to examine the possible benefits of stimulators of osteoblast function to reverse the process. Sodium fluoride is a potent stimulator of osteoblast function by recruitment of osteoblasts[212], and has been found to be effective in small numbers of patients, who were also receiving low doses of vitamin D and calcium[32], with striking increases in trabecular bone volume and osteoid surfaces[65].

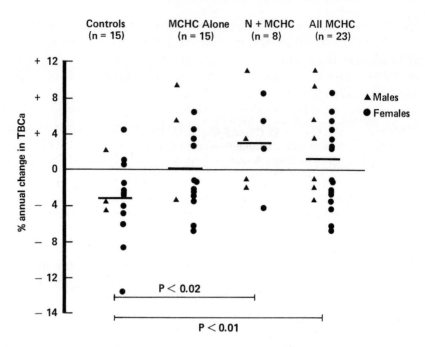

FIGURE 5.5   Percentage annual change in total-body calcium (%TBCa) in controls and corticosteroid-treated patients receiving therapy with calcium (MCHC) alone and nandrolone decanoate plus calcium (N+MCHC), compared with disease controls (from ref. 215, reproduced by kind permission of the publishers, Osteopress ApS, Copenhagen)

The realization that anabolic steroids stimulated osteoblast pro-liferation *in vitro*[213] has led to their use as possible therapies for corticosteroid-induced osteoporosis. Low osteocalcin levels can be normalized by nandrolone decanoate[214] and the same drug has been shown to increase forearm bone mineral density in a small number of patients[19]. In a small study we have recently shown that total bone mass can be significantly increased (by a mean of 2.9% per annum) in patients receiving nandrolone decanoate 50 mg every 3 weeks com-pared with disease controls (Figure 5.5)[214].

The effect on fracture rate of these various possible therapies for corticosteroid-induced osteoporosis has not been systematically studied, and much more work is required to determine whether the favourable effects on bone mass of 25(OH)D, bisphosphonates, calcitonin, sodium fluoride and anabolic steroids can be translated into the ultimate goal of reduced fracture occurrence.

REFERENCES

1. Cushing, H. (1932). The basophil adenomas of the pituitary and their clinical manifestations. *Bull. Johns Hopkins Hosp.,* **50,** 137–95.
2. Howland, W. J., Pugh, D. C. and Sprague, R. G. (1958). Roentgenologic changes in the skeletal system in Cushing's syndrome. *Radiology,* **71,** 69–78.
3. Soffer, L. J., Iannaccone, A. and Gabrilove, J. L. (1961). Cushing's syndrome. A study of fifty patients. *Am. J. Med.,* **30,** 129–46.
4. Kleerkoper, M., Rao, D. S., Matovic, V., Whyte, M. P. and Avioli, L. V. (1979). Endogenous Cushing's disease in two adults presenting with osteopenia as the major clinical manifestation. In Barzell, U. S. (ed.), *Osteoporosis II.* (New York: Grune & Stratton), p. 244.
5. Sprague, R. G., Randall, R. V., Scilassa, R. M., Scholz, D. A., Priestley, J. T., Walters, W. and Bulbulian, A. H. (1956). Cushing's syndrome. A progressive and often fatal disease. *Arch. Intern. Med.,* **98,** 389–98.
6. Ross, E. J. and Linch, D. C. (1982). Cushing's syndrome – killing disease: discriminatory value of signs and symptoms aiding early diagnosis. *Lancet, 2,* 646–9.
7. Urbanic, R. C. and George, J. M. (1981). Cushing's disease – 18 years experience. *Medicine (Baltimore),* **60,** 14–24.
8. Pocock, N. A., Eisman, J. A., Dunstan, C. R., Evans, R. A., Thomas, D. H. and Laila, N. (1987). Recovery from steroid-induced osteoporosis. *Ann. Intern. Med.,* **107,** 319–23.
9. West, T. B., Keck, E., Kohlsdorfer, W. and Kruskemper, H. L. (1983). Bone mineral content by photon absorptiometry in hyperthyroidism and endogenous Cushing's syndrome. *Calcif. Tissue Int.,* **35s,** 270.
10. Genant, H. K., Cann, C. E. and Foul, D. D. (1982). Quantitative computed tomography for assessing vertebral bone mineral. In Dequeker, J. and Johnston, C. C. (eds.), *Non-invasive Bone Measurements* (Oxford: IRL Press), pp. 215–49.
11. Nordin, B. E. C. (1976). Plasma calcium and plasma magnesium homeostasis. In Nordin, B. E. C. (ed.), *Calcium, Phosphate and Magnesium Metabolism* (Edinburgh: Churchill Livingstone), pp. 186–216.
12. Aloia, J. F., Roginsky, M., Ellis, K., Shukla, K. and Cohn, S. (1974). Skeletal metabolism and body composition in Cushing's syndrome. *J. Clin. Endocrinol. Metab.,* **39,** 981–5.
13. Hench, P. S., Kendall, E. C., Slocumb, C. H. and Polley, H. F. (1949). Effect of a hormone of the adrenal cortex (17-hydroxy-11-dehydrocorticosterone: compound E) and of pituitary adrenocorticotrophic hormone on rheumatoid arthritis. *Proc. Mayo Clin.,* **24,** 181–97.
14. Boland, E. W. and Headley, N. E. (1950). Management of rheumatoid arthritis with smaller (maintenance) doses of cortisone acetate. *J. Am. Med. Assoc.,* **144,** 365–72.
15. Curtess, P. H. Jr., Clark, W. S. and Herndon, C. H. (1954). Vertebral fractures resulting from prolonged cortisone and corticotrophin therapy. *J. Am. Med. Assoc.,* **156,** 467–9.

16. Rosenberg, E. F. (1958). Rheumatoid arthritis. Osteoporosis and fractures related to steroid therapy. *Acta Med. Scand., 341s*, 211–24.
17. Virkkunen, M. and Lehtinen, L. (1958). Side effects of corticosteroids. Observations after five years continuous use. *Acta Med. Scand., 341s*, 205–10.
18. Murray, R. O. (1960). Radiological bone changes in Cushing's syndrome and steroid therapy. *Br. J. Radiol., 33*, 1–19.
19. Need, A. G. (1987). Corticosteroids and osteoporosis. *Aust. N.Z. J. Med., 17*, 267–72.
20. Steinbrocker, O., Berkowitz, S. and Carp, S. (1951). ACTH and cortisone as the therapeutic agents in arthritis and some locomotor disorders. *Bull. N.Y. Acad. Med., 27*, 560–76.
21. Arnoldson H. (1958). Long term ACTH and corticosteroid therapy in bronchial asthma. *Acta Allergol., 12* (Suppl. 6), 1–190.
22. Boland, E. W. (1951). Prolonged uninterrupted cortisone therapy in rheumatoid arthritis. *Br. Med. J., 2*, 191–9.
23. Burrage, W. S., Ritchie, A. C., Mansmann, H. C., Irwin, J. W. and Russfield, A. B. (1958). The use of cortisone and hydrocortisone in allergy. *Ann. Intern. Med., 43*, 1001–18.
24. Badley, B. W. D. and Ansell, B. M. (1960). Fractures in Still's disease. *Ann. Rheum. Dis., 19*, 135–41.
25. Guyatt, G. H., Webber, C. E., Mewa, A. A. and Sackett, D. C. (1984). Determining causation – a case study, adreno-corticosteroids and osteoporosis. *J. Chron. Dis., 37*, 343–52.
26. Peck, W. A., Gennari, C., Raisz, L., Meunier, P., Ritz, E., Krane, S., Nuki, G. and Avioli, L. V. (1984). Round table discussion. Corticosteroid and bone. *Calcif. Tissue Int., 36*, 4–7.
27. Als, O. S., Gotfredsen, A. and Christiansen, C. (1985). The effect of glucocorticoids on bone mass in rheumatoid arthritis patients. *Arthritis Rheum., 28*, 369–75.
28. Verstraeten, A. and Dequeker, J. (1986). Vertebral and peripheral bone mineral content in post menopausal patients with rheumatoid arthritis: effect of low dose corticosteroids. *Ann. Rheum. Dis., 45*, 852–7.
29. Nagant de Deuxchaisnes, C., Devogelaer, J. P., Esselinckx, W., Bouchez, B., Depresseux, C., Rombouts-Lindemans, C. and Haux, H. P. (1984). The effect of low dosage glucocorticoids on bone mass in rheumatoid arthritis: a cross-sectional and a longitudinal study using single photon absorptiometry. *Adv. Exp. Med. Biol., 171*, 209–39.
30. Sambrook, P. N., Eisman, J. A., Champion, D., Yeates, M. G. and Pocock, N. A. (1987). Determinants of axial bone loss in rheumatoid arthritis. *Arthritis Rheum., 30*, 721–8.
31. Hahn, T. J. (1978). Corticosteroid-induced osteoporosis. *Arch. Intern. Med., 138*, 882–5.
32. Baylink, D. J. (1983). Glucocorticoid-induced osteoporosis. *N. Engl. J. Med., 309*, 306–8.
33. Saville, P. D. and Karmosh, O. (1967). Osteoporosis of rheumatoid arthritis. Influence of age, sex, and corticosteroids. *Arthritis Rheum., 10*, 423–30.
34. Deding, A., Taigaard, S., Jensen, M. K. and Rodbro, P. (1977). Bone changes during prednisone treatment. *Acta Med. Scand., 202*, 253–5.

35. Cannigia, A., Nuti, R., Lore, F. and Valtimo, A. (1981). Pathophysiology of the adverse effects of glucoactive corticosteroids on calcium metabolism in man. *J. Steroid Biochem.*, **15**, 153–61.

36. Boyd, R. M., Cameron, E. C., McIntosh, H. W. and Walker, V. R. (1974). Measurement of bone mineral content in vivo using photon absorptiometry. *Can. Med. Assoc. J.*, **111**, 1201–5.

37. Hahn, T. J., Boisseau, V. C. and Avioli, L. V. (1974). Effect of chronic corticosteroid administration on diaphyseal and metaphyseal bone mass. *J. Clin. Endocrinol. Metab.*, **39**, 274–82.

38. Gluck, O. S., Murphy, W. A., Hahn, T. J. and Hahn, B. (1981). Bone loss in adults receiving alternate day glucocorticoid therapy. *Arthritis Rheum.*, **24**, 892–8.

39. Dykman, T. R., Haralson, K. M., Gluck, O. S., Murphy, W. A., Teitelbaum, S. L., Hahn, T. J. and Hahn, B. (1984). Effect of oral 1,25-dihydroxyvitamin D and calcium on glucocorticoid-induced osteopenia in patients with rheumatic diseases. *Arthritis Rheum.*, **27**, 1336–43.

40. Adinoff, A. D. and Hollister, J. R. (1983). Steroid induced fractures and bone loss in patients with asthma. *N. Engl. J. Med.*, **309**, 265–8.

41. Rickers, H., Deding, A., Christiansen, C. and Rodbro, P. (1984). Mineral loss in cortical and trabecular bone during high-dose prednisone treatment. *Calcif. Tissue Int.*, **36**, 269–73.

42. Mazess, R. B. (1984). Steroid induced bone loss. *N. Engl. J. Med.*, **310**, 321.

43. Schlenker, R. A. (1976). Percentage of cortical and trabecular bone mineral mass in the radius and ulna. *Am. J. Radiol.*, **126**, 1309–12.

44. Schaadt, O. and Bohr, H. (1982). Loss of bone mineral in axial and peripheral skeleton in ageing, prednisone treatment and osteoporosis. In Dequeker, J. and Johnston, C. C. (eds), *Non-invasive Bone Measurements* (Oxford: IRL Press), pp. 207–14.

45. Schaadt, O. and Bohr, H. (1984). Bone mineral in lumbar spine, femoral neck and femoral shaft measured by dual photon absorptiometry with 153-gadolinium in prednisone treatment. *Adv. Exp. Med. Biol.*, **171**, 201–8.

46. Seeman, E., Wahner, H. W., Offord, K. P., Kumar, R., Johnson, W. J. and Riggs, B. L. (1982). Differential effects of endocrine dysfunction on the axial and appendicular skeleton. *J. Clin. Invest.*, **69**, 1302–9.

47. Zanzi, I., Roginsky, M. S., Ellis, K. J., Blau, S. and Cohn, S. (1976). Skeletal mass in rheumatoid arthritis: a comparison with forearm bone mineral content. *Am. J. Roentgenol. Rad. Ther. Nucl. Med.*, **126**, 1305–6.

48. Reid, D. M., Kennedy, N. S. J., Smith, M. A., Tothill, P. and Nuki, G. (1982). Total body calcium in rheumatoid arthritis: effects of disease activity and corticosteroid treatment. *Br. Med. J.*, **285**, 330–2.

49. Als, O. S., Gotfredsen, A. and Christiansen, C. Relationship between local and total bone mineral in patients with rheumatoid arthritis and normal subjects. *Clin. Rhumatol.*, **2**, 265–71.

50. Kennedy, A. C., Boddy, K., Williams, E. D., Elliot, A. T., Harvey, I., Holloway, I. and Haywood, J. K. (1979). Whole body elemental composition during drug treatment of rheumatoid arthritis: a preliminary study. *Ann. Rheum. Dis.*, **38**, 137–40.

51. Gallagher, J. C., Aaron, J., Horsman, A., Wilkinson, R. and Nordin, B. E. C. (1973). Corticosteroid osteoporosis. *Clin. Endocrinol. Metab.* **2**, 355–68.

52. Reid, D. M. (1984). Bone mass in rheumatic diseases. MD thesis, University of Aberdeen.

53. Reid, D. M., Nicoll, J. J., Brown, N., Tothill, P. and Nuki, G. (1988). Measurement of hand bone mass by single photon absorptiometry in rheumatoid arthritis and asthma: comparison with metacarpal indices. *Clin. Phys. Physiol. Meas.,* **9,** 175–87.

54. Kalla, A. A., Meyers, O. L., Parkyn, N. D. and Kotze, T. (1987). Radiogrammetry in rheumatic disease: Effects of corticosteroid therapy. In Christiansen, C., Johansen, J. S. and Riis, B. J. (eds), *Osteoporosis 1987* (Copenhagen: Osteopress ApS), pp. 1083–4.

55. Greenberger, P. A., Hendrix, R. W., Patterson, R. and Chmiel, J. S. (1982). Bone studies in patients on prolonged systemic corticosteroid treatment for asthma. *Clin. Allergy,* **12,** 363–8.

56. Nicoll, J. J., Smith, M. A., Reid, D., Law, E., Brown, N., Tothill, P. and Nuki, G. (1987). Measurement of hand bone mineral content using single-photon absorptiometry. *Phys. Med. Biol.,* **32,** 697–706.

57. Ruegsegger, P., Medici, T. C. and Anliker, M. (1983). Corticosteroid induced bone loss. A longitudinal study using computed tomography. *Eur. J. Clin. Pharmacol.,* **25,** 615–20.

58. Fujii, Y., Tsunenari, T., Tsutsumi, M., Fukase, M., Yoshimoto, Y. and Fujita, T. (1987). Quantitative computed tomography of lumbar vertebrae in Japanese patients with steroid-induced osteopenia. In Christiansen, C., Johnansen, J. S. and Riis, B. J. (eds), *Osteoporosis 1987* (Copenhagen: Osteopress ApS), pp. 1065–7.

59. Ortoft, G. and Oxlund, H. (1987). The effect of glucocorticoids on the strength of rat cortical bone. In Christiansen, C., Johansen, J. S. and Riis, B. J. (eds) *Osteoporosis 1987* (Copenhagen: Osteopress ApS), pp. 1070–1.

60. Peck, W. A. (1984). The effects of glucocorticoids on bone cell metabolism and function. *Adv. Exp. Med. Biol.,* **171,** 111–9.

61. Birkenhager, J. C., van der Heul, R. O., Smeenk, D., van der Sluys, P., Veer, J. and van Seters, A. P. (1967). Bone changes associated with glucocorticoid excess. *Proc. R. Soc. Med.,* **60,** 1134–6.

62. Hahn, T. J., Halstead, L. R., Teitelbaum, S. L. and Hahn, B. H. (1979). Altered mineral metabolism in gluco-corticoid induced osteopenia. *J. Clin. Invest.,* **64,** 655–65.

63. Jowsey, J. and Riggs, B. L. (1970). Bone formation in hypercortisonism. *Acta Endocrinol.,* **63,** 21–8.

64. Bressot, C., Meunier, P. J., Chapuy, M. C., Lejeune, E., Edouard, C. and Darby, A. J. (1979). Histomorphometric profile, pathophysiology and reversibility of corticosteroid induced osteoporosis. *Metab. Bone Dis. Relat. Res.,* **1,** 303–11.

65. Meunier, P. J., Dempster, D. W., Edouard, C., Chapuy, M. C., Arlot, M. and Charhon, S. (1984). Bone histomorphometry in corticosteroid-induced osteoporosis and Cushing's syndrome. *Adv. Exp. Med. Biol.,* **171,** 191–200.

66. Jee, W. S. S. and Clark, I. (1981). Glucocorticoid-induced osteoporosis. In DeLuca, H. F., Frost, H. M., Jee, W. S. S., Johnston, C. C. and Parfitt, A. M. (eds), *Osteoporosis: Recent Advances in Pathogenesis and Treatment* (Baltimore: University Park Press), pp. 331–42.

67. Frost, H. M. and Villaneuva, A. R. (1961). Human osteoblastic activity. III. The

effect of cortisone on lamellar osteoblastic activity. *Henry Ford Hosp. Med. Bull.,* **9.** 91–7.

68. Klein, D. C. and Raisz, L. G. (1970). Prostaglandins. Stimulation of bone resorption in tissue culture. *Endocrinology,* **86,** 1436–40.
69. Dempster, D. W., Arlot, M. and Meunier, P. J. (1983). Mean wall thickness and formation periods of trabecular bone packets in corticosteroid-induced osteoporosis. *Calcif. Tissue Int.,* **33,** 410–7.
70. Hahn, T. J. (1980). Drug induced disorders of vitamin D and mineral metabolism. *Clin. Endocrinol. Metab.,* **9,** 107–29.
71. Teitelbaum, S. L. and Kahn, T. J. (1980). Mononuclear phagocytes, osteoclasts and bone resorption. *Miner. Electrolyte. Metab.,* **3,** 2–7.
72. Teitelbaum, S. L., Stewart, C. C. and Kahn, A. J. (1979). Rodent macrophages as bone resorbing cells. *Calcif. Tissue Int.,* **27,** 255–61.
73. Teitelbaum, S. L., Malone, J. D. and Kahn, A. J. (1981). Glucocorticoid enhancement of bone resorption by rat peritoneal macrophages in vitro. *Endocrinology,* **108,** 795–9.
74. Tashjian, A. H. Jr., Hohmann, E. L., Antoniades, H. N. and Levine, L. (1982). Platelet-derived growth factor stimulates bone resorption via a prostaglandin-mediated mechanism. *Endocrinology,* **111,** 118–24.
75. Stern, P. H. Inhibition by steroids of parathyroid hormone induced Ca^{45} release from embryonic rat bone *in vitro.* (1969). *J. Pharmacol. Exp. Ther.,* **168,** 211–7.
76. Raisz, L. G., Trummel, C. L., Wener, J. A. and Simmons, H. (1972). Effect of glucocorticoids on bone resorption in tissue culture. *Endocrinology,* **90,** 961–7.
77. Imbimbo, C., Malone, J. D. and Kahn, A. J. (1984). Glucocorticoids and bone resorption. *Adv. Exp. Med. Biol.,* **171,** 121–9.
78. Kimberg, D. V., Baery, R. D., Gershon, E. and Graudusius, R. T. (1971). Effect of cortisone treatment on the active transport of calcium by the small intestine. *J. Clin. Invest.,* **50,** 1309–21.
79. Hahn, T. J., Halstead, L. R. and Baron, D. T. (1981). Effects of short term glucocorticoid administration on intestinal calcium absorption and circulating vitamin D metabolite concentrations in man. *J. Clin. Endocrinol. Metab.,* **52,** 111–5.
80. Klein, R. G., Arnaud, S. B., Gallagher, J. C., DeLuca, H. F. and Riggs, B. L. (1977). Intestinal calcium absorption in exogenous hypercortisonism. *J. Clin. Invest.,* **60,** 253–9.
81. Crilly, R. G., Brown, W., Peacock, M. and Nordin, B. E. C. (1982). Malabsorption of calcium in steroid induced osteoporosis. *Clin. Sci.,* **62,** 41p.
82. Favus, M. J. Pathophysiology of gluco-corticoid induced osteoporosis and the alterations of parathyroid and vitamin D function. In Christiansen, C., Johansen, J. S. and Riis, B. J. (eds), *Osteoporosis 1987* (Copenhagen: Osteopress ApS), pp. 1028–32.
83. Crilly, R. G., Peacock, M., Taylor, G. A. and Nordin, B. E. C. (1981). Effect of corticosteroid therapy on plasma 1,25-dihydroxy-vitamin D levels. *Clin. Sci.,* **60,** 26p.
84. Chesney, R. W., Mazess, R. B., Hamstra, A. J., DeLuca, H. F. and O'Reagan, S. (1978). Reduction of serum 1,25 dihydroxyvitamin D_3 in children receiving glucocorticoids. *Lancet,* **2,** 1123–5.
85. Seeman, E., Kumar, R., Hunder, G. G., Scott, M., Heath, H. III and Riggs,

B. L. (1980). Production, degradation and circulating levels of 1,25-dihydroxyvitamin D in health and in glucocorticoid excess. *J. Clin. Invest.*, **66**, 664–9.

86. Luengo, M., Picado, C., Guanabens, N., Rivera, F., Piera, C., Monsterat, J. M. and Augusti-Vidal, A. (1987). Effects of chronic corticosteroid therapy on mineral metabolic and intestinal calcium absorption in corticodependent asthmatics. In Christiansen, C., Johansen, J. S. and Riis, B. J. (eds), *Osteoporosis 1987* (Copenhagen: Osteopress ApS), pp. 1051–2.

87. Hahn, T. J., Halstead, L. R. and Haddad, J. G. (1977). Serum 25-hydroxyvitamin D concentrations in patients receiving corticosteroid therapy. *J. Clin. Lab. Med.*, **90**, 399–404.

88. Avioli, L. V., Birge, S. J. and Lee, S. W. (1968). Effects of vitamin D metabolism in man. *J. Clin. Endocrinol. Metab.*, **28**, 1341–6.

89. Gennari, C., Bernini, M., Nardi, P., Fusi, L., Francini, G., Nami, R., Montagnani, M., Imbimbo, B. and Avioli, L. (1983). Glucocorticoids. Radiocalcium and radiophosphate absorption in man. In Dixon, A. St J., Russell, R. G. G. and Stamp, T. C. B. (eds), *Osteoporosis: A Multidisciplinary Problem.* Royal Society of Medicine Congress and Symposium Series No. 55. (London: Academic Press and Royal Society of Medicine), pp. 75–80.

90. Pressley, L. and Funder, J. W. (1975). Glucocorticoid and mineralocorticoid receptors in gut mucosa. *Endocrinology*, **97**, 588–96.

91. Holdsworth, C. D. (1975). Calcium absorption in man. In McColl,I. and Sladen, G. E. (eds), *Intestinal Absorption in Man* (London: Academic Press), pp. 223–62.

92. Harrison, H. E. and Harrison, H. C. (1960). Transfer of ^{47}Ca across the intestinal walls in vitro in relation to the action of vitamin D and cortisol. *Am. J. Physiol.*, **179**, 265–71.

93. Favus, M. J., Walting, M. W. and Kimberg, D. V. (1973). Effects of 1,25-dihydroxycholecalciferol on intestinal calcium transport in cortisone-treated rats. *J. Clin. Invest.*, **52**, 1680–5.

94. Chan, S. D. H., Chiu, D. K. H. and Atkins, D. (1984). Mechanism of the regulation of the 1,25-dihydroxyvitamin D receptor in the rat jejunum by glucocorticoids. *J. Endocrinol.*, **103**, 295–30.

95. Korkor, A. B., Kuchibotla, J., Arrieh, M. Gray, R. W. and Gleason, W. A. Jr. (1985). The effects of chronic prednisone administration on intestinal receptors for 1,25-dihydroxyvitamin D_3 in the dog. *Endocrinology*, **117**, 2267–73.

96. Raisz, L. G., Trummel, C. L., Holick, M. F. and DeLuca, H. F. (1972). 1,25 Dihydroxycholecalciferol: a potent stimulator of bone resorption in tissue culture. *Science,* **175**, 768–9.

97. Narbaitz, R., Stumpf, W. E., Sar, M., Huang, S. and DeLuca, H. F. (1983). Autoradiographic localization of target cells for 1 alpha,25-dihydroxyvitamin D_3 in bones from fetal rats. *Calcif. Tissue Int.*, **35**, 177–82.

98. Gennari, C. and Civitelli, R. (1986). Glucocorticoid-induced osteoporosis. *Clin. Rheum. Dis.*, **12**, 637–54.

99. Wajchenberg, B. L., Pereira, V. G., Kieffer, J. and Uric, S. (1969). Effect of dexamethasone on calcium metabolism and ^{47}Ca kinetics in normal subjects. *Acta Endocrinol.*, **61**, 173–92.

100. Suzuki, Y., Ichikawa, Y., Saito, E. and Homma, M. (1983). Importance of increased calcium excretion in the development of secondary hyper-

parathyroidism of patients under glucocorticoid therapy. *Metabolism*, **32,** 151–6.

101. Au, W. Y. W. (1976). Cortisol stimulation of parathyroid hormone secretion by rat parathyroid glands in organ culture. *Science,* **193,** 1015–7.

102. Fucik, R. F., Kukreja, S. C., Hargis, G. K., Bowser, E. N., Henderson, W. J. and Williams, G. A. (1975). Effects of glucocorticoids on function of the parathyroid glands in man. *J. Clin. Endocrinol. Metab.,* **40,** 152–5.

103. Lukert, B. P. and Adams, J. S. (1976). Calcium and phosphorus homeostasis in man: Effect of corticosteroids. *Arch. Int. Med.,* **136,** 1249–53.

104. Gennari, C., Imbimbo, B., Montagnani, M., Bernini, M., Nardi, P. and Avioli, L. V. (1984). Effects of prednisone and deflazacort on mineral metabolism and parathyroid hormone activity in humans. *Calcif. Tissue Int.,* **36,** 245–52.

105. Slovik, D. M., Neer, R. M., Ohman, J. L., Lowell, F. C., Clark, M. B., Segre, G. V. and Potts, J. T. Jr. (1980). Parathyroid hormone and 25-hydroxyvitamin D levels in glucocorticoid-treated patients. *Clin. Endocrinol.,* **12,** 243–8.

106. Jee, W. S. S., Park, H. Z., Roberts, W. E. and Kenner, G. H. (1970). Corticosteroid and bone. *Am. J. Anat.,* **129,** 477–81.

107. Rodan, G. A., and Martin T. J. (1981). Role of osteoblasts in hormonal control of bone resorption – a hypothesis. *Calcif. Tissue Int.,* **33,** 349–51.

108. Chen, T. L. and Feldman, D. (1979). Glucorticoid receptors and actions in sub populations of cultured rat bone cells. Mechanism of dexamethasone potentiation of parathyroid hormone-stimulated cyclic AMP production. *J. Clin. Invest.,* **63,** 750–8.

109. Feldman, D. and Kirshnan, A. V. (1987). Glucocorticoid effects on calcium metabolism and bone in the development of osteopenia. In Christiansen, C., Johansen, J. S. and Riis, B. J. (eds), *Osteoporosis 1987* (Copenhagen: Osteopress ApS), pp. 1006–13.

110. Lo Cascio, V., Adami, S., Avioli, L. V., Cominacini, L., Galvanini, G., Gennari, C., Imbimbo, B. and Scuro, L. A. (1982). Suppressive effect of chronic glucocorticoid treatment on circulating calcitonin in man. *Calcif. Tissue Int.,* **34,** 309–10.

111. Thompson, J. S., Palmieri, G. M. A., Eliel, L. P. and Crawford, R. L. (1972). The effect of porcine calcitonin on osteoporosis induced by adrenal corticosteroids. *J. Bone Joint Surg. [Am.],* **54,** 1490–500.

112. Crilly, R. G., Marshall, D. H. and Nordin, B. E. C. (1979). Metabolic effects of corticosteroid therapy in post-menopausal women. *J. Steroid Biochem.,* **11,** 429–33.

113. Nordin, B. E. C., Robertson, A. and Seamark, R. F. (1985). The relation between calcium absorption, serum dehydroepiandrosterone and vertebral mineral density in postmenopausal women. *J. Clin. Endocrinol. Metab.,* **60,** 651–7.

114. Danisova, A., Sebokova, E. and Kolena, J. (1987). Effect of corticosteroids on estradiol and testosterone secretion by granulosa cells in culture. *Exp. Clin. Endocrinol.,* **89,** 165–73.

115. Strewler, G. J. (1987). Physiology and biochemistry of glucocorticoid action. In Christiansen, C., Johansen, J. S. and Riis, B. J. (eds), *Osteoporosis 1987* (Copenhagen: Osteopress ApS), pp. 998–1005.

116. Gowen, M., Wood, D. D., Ihrie, E. J., McGuire, M. K. B. and Russell, R. G. G. (1983). An interleukin 1 like factor stimulates bone resorption in vitro. *Nature,* **306,** 378–80.

117. Bertolini, D. R., Nedwin, G. E., Bringman, T. S., Smith, D. D. and Mundy, G. R. (1986). Stimulation of bone resorption and inhibition of bone formation in vitro by human tumour necrosis factor. *Nature*, **319**, 516–8.

118. Lerner, U. H., Jones, I. L. and Gustafson, G. T. (1987). Bradykinin, a new potential mediator of inflammation-induced bone resorption. *Arthritis Rheum.*, **30**, 530–40.

119. Hahn, T. J., Halstead, L. R., Strates, B., Imbimbo, B. and Baron, D. T. (1979). Comparison of subacute effects of oxazacort and prednisone on mineral metabolism in man. *Calcif. Tissue Int.*, **31**, 109–15.

120. Braun, J. J., Birkenhager-Frenkel, D. H., Rietveld, J. R., Juttmann, J. R., Visser, T. J. and Birkenhager, J. C. (1983). Influence of $1\alpha(OH)D_3$ administration on bone and bone mineral metabolism in patients on glucocorticoid treatment; a double blind controlled study. *Clin. Endocrinol.*, **19**, 165–73.

121. Nordin, B. E. C., Marshall, D. H., Francis, R. M. and Crilly, R. G. (1981). The effects of sex steroid and corticosteroid hormones on bone. *J. Steroid Biochem.*, **15**, 171–4.

122. Als, O. S., Christiansen, C. and Hellesen, C. (1984). Prevalence of decreased bone mass in rheumatoid arthritis: Relation to anti-inflammatory treatment. *Clin. Rheumatol.*, **3**, 201–8.

123. Chen, T. L., Aronow, L. and Feldman, D. (1977). Glucocorticoid receptors and inhibition of bone cell growth in primary culture. *Endocrinology*, **100**, 619–28.

124. Manolagas, S. C. and Anderson, D. C. (1978). Detection of high affinity glucocorticoid binding in rat bone. *J. Endocrinol.*, **76**, 377–80.

125. Haussler, M. R., Manolagas, S. C. and Deftos, L. J. (1980). Glucocorticoid receptor in clonal osteosarcoma cell lines: a novel system for investigating bone active hormones. *Biochem. Biophys. Res. Commun.*, **94**, 373–80.

126. Cannalis, E. (1983). Effect of glucocorticoids on type I collagen synthesis, alkaline phosphatase activity and deoxyribonucleic acid content in cultured rat calvariae. *Endocrinology*, **112**, 931–9.

127. Raisz, L. and Chyun, Y. S. (1984). Glucocorticoids and bone matrix formation. *Adv. Exp. Med. Biol.*, **171**, 131–6.

128. Chyun, Y. S. and Raisz, L. G. (1982). Opposing effects of prostaglandin E2 and cortisol on bone growth in organ culture. *Clin. Res.*, **30**, 387A.

129. Peck, W. A., Brandt, J. and Miller, I. (1967). Hydrocortisone-induced inhibition of protein synthesis and uridine incorporation in isolated bone cells in vitro. *Proc. Natl. Acad. Sci.*, **57**, 1599–606.

130. Choe, J., Stern, P. and Feldman, D. (1977). Receptor mediated glucocorticoid inhibition of protein synthesis in isolated bone cells. *J. Steroid Biochem.*, **9**, 265–71.

131. Nishimoto, S. K. and Price, P. A. (1979). Proof that the carboxyglutamic acid-containing bone protein is synthesised in calf bone. Comparative synthesis rate and effect of coumadine on synthesis. *J. Biol. Chem.*, **254**, 437–41.

132. Beresford, J. N., Gallagher, J. A., Poser, J. W. and Russell, R. G. G. (1984). Production of osteocalcin by human bone cells in vitro. Effects of $1,25(OH)_2D_3$, parathyroid hormone and glucocorticoids. *Metab. Bone Dis. Relat. Res.*, **5**, 229–34.

133. Reid, I. R., Chapman, G. E., Fraser, T. R. C., Davies, A. D., Surus, A. S., Meyer, J., Huq, N. L. and Ibbertson, H. K. (1986). Low serum osteocalcin levels in glucocorticoid–treated asthmatics. *J. Clin. Endocrinol. Metab.*, **62**, 379–83.

134. Delmas, P. D. (1987). Clinical applications of serum GLA-protein (osteocalcin) assays in metabolic bone diseases. In Christiansen, C., Johansen, J. S. and Riis, B. J. (eds), *Osteoporosis 1987* (Copenhagen: Osteopress ApS), pp. 664–671.

135. Lukert, B. P., Higgins, J. C. and Stoskopf, M. (1986). Serum osteocalcin is increased in patients with hyperthyroidism and decreased in patients receiving glucocorticoids. *J. Clin. Endocrinol. Metab.*, **62**, 1056–8.

136. Weisman, W. H., Orth, R. W., Catherwood, B. D., Manolagas, S. C. and Deftos, L. J. (1986). Measures of bone loss in rheumatoid arthritis. *Arch. Intern. Med.*, **146**, 701–4.

137. Ekenstam, E. A. F., Ljunghall, S. and Hallgren, R. (1986). Serum osteocalcin in rheumatoid arthritis and other inflammatory arthritides: relation between inflammatory activity and the effect of glucocorticoids and remission inducing drugs. *Ann. Rheum. Dis.*, **45**, 484–90.

138. Chen, T. L., Cone, C. M., Morey-Holton, E. and Feldman, D. (1983). $1\alpha,25$-Dihydroxyvitamin D_3 receptors in cultured rat osteoclast-like cells. *J. Biol. Chem.*, **258**, 4350–8.

139. Chen, T. L., Cone, C. M., Morey-Holton, E. and Feldman, D. (1982). Glucocorticoid regulation of $1,25(OH)_2$-vitamin D_3 receptors in cultured mouse bone cells. *J. Biol. Chem.*, **257**, 13564–9.

140. Beresford, J. N., Gallagher, J. A. and Russell, R. G. G. (1986). 1,25 Dihydroxyvitamin D_3 and human bone derived cells in vitro. Effects on alkaline phosphatase, type I collagen and proliferation. *Endocrinology*, **119**, 1776–85.

141. McSheehy, P. M. J. and Chambers, T. J. (1987). 1,25 Dihydroxyvitamin D_3 stimulates osteoblastic cells to release a soluble factor that increases osteoclastic bone resorption. *J. Clin. Invest.*, **80**, 425–9.

142. Jowell, P. S., Epstein, S., Fallon, M. D., Reinhardt, T. A. and Ismail, F. (1987). 1,25-Dihydroxyvitamin D_3 modulates glucocorticoid-induced alteration in serum GLA protein and bone histomorphometry. *Endocrinology*, **120**, 531–8.

143. MacAdams, M. R., White, R. H. and Chipps, B. E. (1986). Reduction of serum testosterone levels during chronic glucocorticoid therapy, *Ann. Intern. Med.*, **104**, 648–51.

144. Lehman, W. L., Solomons, C. C. and Hollister, J. R. (1984). Calmodulin activity in corticosteroid-induced osteopenia. *Clin. Orthop.*, **187**, 300–7.

145. Peretz, A., Neve, J., Vertongen, F., Famaey, J. P. and Molle, L. (1987). Selenium status in relation to clinical variables and corticosteroid treatment in rheumatoid arthritis. *J. Rheumatol.*, **14**, 1104–7.

146. Elsasser, U., Wilkins, B., Hesp, R., Thurnham, D. I., Reeve, J. and Ansell, B. M. (1982). Bone rarefaction and crush fractures in juvenile chronic arthritis. *Arch. Dis. Child.*, **57**, 377–80.

147. Hahn, B. H., Dykman, T., Lewis-Stevens, D., Haralson, K., Murphy, W. and Hahn, T. J. (1981). Incidence of bone fractures in rheumatic disease patients treated with and without glucocorticoids. *Clin. Res.*, **29**, 782A.

148. Luengo, M., Picado, C., Guanbens, N., Del Rio, L., Brancos, M. A. and Montserrat, J. M. (1987). Bone loss in chronic corticodependent asthma. In Christiansen, C., Johansen, J. S. and Riis, B. J. (eds), *Osteoporosis 1987* (Copenhagen: Osteopress ApS), pp. 1068–9.

149. Dykman, T. R., Gluck, O. S., Murphy, W. A., Hahn, T. J. and Hahn, B. H. (1985). Evaluation of factors associated with glucocorticoid induced osteopenia

in patients with rheumatic diseases. *Arthritis Rheum.*, **28**, 361–8.

150. Paganini-Hill, A., Ross, R. K., Gerkins, V. R., Henderson, B. E., Arthur, M. and Mack, T. M. (1981). Menopausal estrogen therapy and hip fractures. *Ann. Intern. Med.*, **95**, 28–31.

151. Gallagher, J. C., Melton, L. J. and Riggs, B. L. (1980). Examination of prevalence rates of possible risk factors in a population with a fracture of the proximal femur. *Clin. Orthop. Rel. Res.*, **153**, 158–65.

152. Currie, A. L., Reid, D. M., Brown, N. and Nuki, G. (1986). An epidemiological study of fracture of the neck of femur in the general population and in patients with rheumatoid arthritis. *Br. J. Rheumatol.*, **25**, 121.

153. Cohn, S. H., Ellis, K. J., Wallach, S., Zanzi, I., Atkins, H. L. and Alloia, J. F. (1974). Absolute and relative deficit in total skeletal calcium and radial bone mineral in osteoporosis. *J. Nucl. Med.*, **15**, 428–35.

154. Eastell, R., Kennedy, N. S. J., Smith, M. A., Simpson, J. D., Strong, J. A. and Tothill, P. (1983). The assessment of postmenopausal osteoporosis by total body neutron activation analysis. *Metab. Bone Dis. Relat. Res.*, **5**, 65–7.

155. Ott, S. M., Murano, R., Lewellen, T. K., Nelp, W. B. and Chestnut, C. H. (1983). Total body calcium by neutron activation analysis in normals and osteoporotic populations: a discriminator of significant bone loss. *J. Lab. Clin. Med.*, **102**, 637–45.

156. Lachmann, E. (1955). Osteoporosis: The potentialities and limitations of its roentgenologic diagnosis. *Am. J. Roentgenol. Rad. Ther. Nucl. Med.*, **74**, 712–5.

157. Reifenstein, E. C. J. (1957). Definitions, terminology and classification of metabolic bone disorders. *Clin. Orthop.*, **9**, 30–44.

158. Maladague, B., Malghem, J. and Nagant de Deuxchaisnes, C. (1984). Radiological aspects of glucocorticoid-induced bone disease. *Adv. Exp. Med. Biol.*, **171**, 155–90.

159. Reid, D. M., Kennedy, N. S. J., Nicoll, J., Smith, M. A., Tothill, P. and Nuki, G. (1986). Total and peripheral bone mass in patients with psoriatic arthritis and rheumatoid arthritis. *Clin. Rheumatol.*, **5**, 372–8.

160. Sambrook, P. N., Eisman, J. A., Yeates, M. G., Pocock, N. A., Eberl, S. and Champion, G. D. (1986). Osteoporosis in rheumatoid arthritis: Safety of low dose corticosteroids. *Ann. Rheum. Dis.*, **45**, 950–3.

161. Tothill, P., Pye, D., Nicoll, J. J., Smith, M. A., Reid, D. M. and Nuki, G. (1987). Spine bone mineral in rheumatoid arthritis and asthma: Effects of corticosteroids and comparison with total body calcium. In Christiansen, C., Johansen, J. S. and Riis, B. J. (eds). *Osteoporosis 1987* (Copenhagen: Osteopress ApS), pp. 664–71.

162. Mueller, M. N. (1976). Effects of corticosteroids on bone mineral in rheumatoid arthritis and asthma. *Am. J. Roentgenol.*, **126**, 1300.

163. Reid, D. M., Nicoll, J., Kennedy, N. S. J., Smith, M. A., Tothill, P., Thompson, A. and Nuki, G. (1984). Bone mass in rheumatoid arthritis, polymyalgia rheumatica and asthma: disease determines susceptibility to corticosteroid induced osteoporosis. In Christiansen, C., Arnaud, C. D., Nordin, B. E. C., Parfitt, A. M., Peck, W. A. and Riggs, B. L. (eds) *Osteoporosis*. (Copenhagen: Department of Clinical Chemistry, Glostrup Hospital), pp. 217–18.

164. Reid, D. M., Nicoll, J. J., Smith, M. A., Higgins, B., Tothill, P. and Nuki, G. (1986). Corticosteroids and bone mass in asthma: comparisons with rheumatoid arthritis and polymyalgia rheumatica. *Br. Med. J.*, **293**, 1463–6.

165. Woolf, A. D., Amin, S. N. and Ring, F. (1987). Corticosteroids and bone mass in polymyalgia rheumatica. In Christiansen, C., Johansen, J. S. and Riis, B. J. (eds), *Osteoporosis 1987*. (Copenhagen: Osteopress ApS), pp. 1062–4.

166. Doherty, S. M. and Grainger, D. (1988). Broadband ultrasound attenuation of the os calcis in patients with known osteoporosis or rheumatic diseases. *Clin. Phys. Physiol. Meas.,* **9,** 185.

167. Taggart, A. J., Astbury, C., Dixon, J. S. and Bird, H. A. (1986). Prednisolone pharmacokinetics in patients with rheumatoid arthritis, polymyalgia rheumatica and asthma. *Clin. Rheumatol.,* **5,** 327–31.

168. Reifenstein, E. C. (1958). Control of corticoid-induced protein depletion and osteoporosis by anabolic steroid therapy. *Metabolism,* **7,** 78–89.

169. Duncan, H. (1972). Osteoporosis in rheumatoid arthritis and corticosteroid induced osteoporosis. *Orthop. Clin. N. Am.,* **3,** 571–83.

170. Klein, M., Villanueva, A. R. and Frost, H. M. (1965). A quantitative histological study of rib from 18 patients treated with adrenal corticosteroids. *Acta Orthop. Scand.,* **35,** 171–84.

171. Rickers, H., Deding, A., Christiansen, C., Rodro, P. and Naestoft, J. (1982). Corticosteroid-induced osteopenia and vitamin D metabolism. Effect of vitamin D_2, calcium, phosphate and sodium fluoride administration. *Clin. Endocrinol.,* **16,** 409–15.

172. Reid, D. M., Kennedy, N. S. J., Smith, M. A., Nicoll, J., Brown, N., Tothill, P. and Nuki, G. (1986). Bone loss in rheumatoid arthritis and primary generalised osteoarthrosis: effects of corticosteroids, suppressive antirheumatic drugs and calcium supplements. *Br. J. Rheumatol.,* **25,** 253–9.

173. Hosking, D. J. and Chamberlain, M. J. (1973). Osteoporosis and long-term corticosteroid therapy. *Br. Med. J.,* **3,** 125–7.

174. Bjelle, A. O. and Nilsson, B. E. (1971). The relationship between radiological changes and osteoporosis of the hand in rheumatoid arthritis. *Arthritis Rheum.,* **14,** 646–9.

175. Crilly, R. G., Marshall, D. H., Horsman, A., Nordin, B. E. C. and Peacock, M. (1983). Corticosteroid osteoporosis. In Dixon, A. St. J., Russell, R. G. G. and Stamp, T. C. B. (eds), *Osteoporosis. A Multidisciplinary Problem.* Royal Society of Medicine Congress and Symposium Series No. 55 (London: Academic Press Inc. and Royal Society of Medicine), pp. 153–9.

176. Lo Cascio, V., Bonucci, E., Imbimbo, B., Ballanti, P., Tartarotti, D., Galvanni, G., Fuccella, L. and Adami, S. (1984). Bone loss after glucocorticoid therapy. *Calcif. Tissue Int.,* **36,** 435–8.

177. Lo Cascio, V., Bonucci, E., Ballanti, P., Adami, S., Rossini, M., Imbimbo, B., Bertoldo, F. and Della Rocca, C. (1987). Glucocorticoid osteoporosis: a longitudinal study. In Christiansen, C., Johansen, J. S. and Riis, B. J. (eds), *Osteoporosis 1987* (Copenhagen: Osteopress ApS), pp. 1062–4.

178. Reid, D. M., Nicoll, J. J., Brown, N., Smith, M. A., Tothill, P. and Nuki, G. (1985). Bone mass in corticosteroid treated patients with rheumatoid arthritis, asthma and polymyalgia rheumatica. *Scott. Med. J.,* **30,** 54–5.

179. Hajiroussou, V. J. and Webley, M. (1984). Prolonged low-dose corticosteroid therapy and osteoporosis in rheumatoid arthritis. *Ann. Rheum. Dis.,* **43,** 24–7.

180. Harris, E. D., Emkey, R. D., Nichols, J. E. and Newberg, A. (1983). Low dose

prednisolone therapy in rheumatoid arthritis: a double blind study. *J. Rheumatol.*, **10**, 713–21.

181. Zerwekh, J. E., Emkey, R. D. and Harris, E. D. (1984). Low-dose prednisone therapy in rheumatoid arthritis: effect on vitamin D metabolism. *Arthritis Rheum.*, **27**, 1050–2.

182. Lund, B., Storm, T. L., Lund, B., Melsen, F., Mosekilde, L., Andersen, R. B., Egmose, C. and Sorensen, O. H. (1985). Bone mineral loss, bone histomorphometry and vitamin D metabolism in patients with rheumatoid arthritis on long-term glucocorticoid treatment. *Clin. Rheumatol.*, **4**, 143–9.

183. Tannebaum, H. (1984). Osteopenia in rheumatology practice: Pathogenesis and therapy. *Semin. Arthritis Rheum.*, **13**, 337–48.

184. West, H. F. (1962). Ten years of ACTH therapy. *Ann. Rheum. Dis.*, **21**, 263–71.

185. Treadwell, B. L. J., Sever, E. D., Savage, O. and Copeman, W. S. C. (1964). Side effects of long term treatment with corticosteroids and corticotrophin. *Lancet*, **1**, 1121–3.

186. Bijlsma, J. W. J., Duursma, S. A. and Huber-Bruning, O. (1986). Bone metabolism during methylprednisolone pulse therapy in rheumatoid arthritis. *Ann. Rheum. Dis.*, **45**, 757–60.

187. Bijlsma, J. W. J., Duursma, S. A., Bosch, R., Raymakers, J. A. and Huber-Bruning, O. (1988). Acute changes in calcium and bone metabolism during methylprednisolone pulse therapy in rheumatoid arthritis. *Br. J. Rheumatol.*, **27**, 215–9.

188. Egsmose, C., Lund, B., Hansen, T. J., Dickmeiss, E., Gerstott, J., Hansen, T. I., Jans, H. and Lorenzen, I. (1987) Effect of mega-dose methylprednisolone in rheumatoid arthritis. In Christiansen, C., Johansen, J. S. and Riis, B. J. (eds), *Osteoporosis 1987* (Copenhagen: Osteopress ApS), pp. 1062–4.

189. Liebling, M. R., Leib, E., McLaughlin, K., Blocka, K., Furst, D. E., Nyman, K. and Paulus, E. (1981). Pulse methylprednisolone in rheumatoid arthritis. *Ann. Intern. Med.*, **94**, 21–6.

190. Anonymous (1984). High-dose corticosteroid inhalers for asthma [Editorial]. *Lancet*, **2**, 23.

191. Jacobson, M. E. (1971). The rationale of alternate-day corticosteroid therapy. *Postgrad. Med.*, **49**, 181–6.

192. Morris, H. G. (1975). Growth and skeletal maturation in asthmatic children: effect of corticosteroid treatment. *Pediat. Res.*, **9**, 579–83.

193. Nilsen, K. H., Jayson, M. I. V. and Dixon, A. St. J. (1978). Microcrystalline calcium hydroxyapatite compound in corticosteroid-treated rheumatoid patients: a controlled study. *Br. Med. J.*, **2**, 1124.

194. Reid, I. R. and Ibbertson, H. K. (1986). Calcium supplementation in the prevention of steroid-induced osteoporosis. *Am. J. Clin. Nutr.*, **44**, 287–90.

195. Robin, J. C. and Ambrus, J. L. (1982). Studies on osteoporosis. IX. Effect of fluoride on steroid induced osteoporosis. *Res. Comm. Chem. Path. Pharmacol.*, **37**, 453–61.

196. Robin, J. C. and Ambrus, J. L. (1982). Studies on osteoporosis VIII. Effect of estrogen on steroid induced osteoporosis. *J. Med. Clin. Exp. Theor.*, **13**, 453–63.

197. Lindgren, J. U. and DeLuca, H. F. (1983). Oral 1,25(OH)$_2$D$_3$ – an effective prophylactic treatment for glucocorticoid osteopenia in rats. *Calcif. Tissue Int.*, **35**, 107–10.

198. Lindgren, J. U., Merchant, C. R. and DeLuca, H. F. (1982). Effect of 1,25 dihydroxyvitamin D_3 on osteopenia induced by prednisolone in adult rats. *Calcif. Tissue Int.*, **34**, 253–7.
199. Lindgren, J. U., DeLuca, H. F. and Mazess, R. B. (1984). Effects of $1,25(OH)_2D_3$ on bone tissue in the rabbit: studies on fracture healing, disuse osteoporosis and prednisone osteoporosis. *Calcif. Tissue Int.*, **36**, 591–5.
200. Lindenhayn, K., Trzenschik, K., Buhler, G. and Wegner, G. (1982). On the action of prednisolone and ethane-1-hydroxy-1,1-diphosphonate (EHDP) on rabbit bone. *Exp. Pathol.*, **21**, 157–64.
201. Avioli, L. (1987). Osteoporosis in rheumatoid arthritis. *Arthritis Rheum.*, **30**, 830–1.
202. Imbimbo, B., Tuzi, T., Porzio, F. and Schianetti, L. (1984). Clinical equivalence of a new glucocorticoid, deflazacort and prednisone in rheumatoid arthritis and S.L.E. patients. *Adv. Exp. Med. Biol.*, **171**, 241–56.
203. Hahn, B. H., Pletscha, L. S. and Muniain, M. (1981). Immunosuppressive effects of a new glucocorticoid with bone-sparing and carbohydrate-sparing properties: comparison with prednisone. *J. Rheumatol.*, **8**, 783–90.
204. Lund, B., Petersen, J. G., Egsmose, C. and Lund, B. (1984). In vitro evidence of the calcium sparing effect of deflazacort. *Adv. Exp. Med. Biol.*, **171**, 149–54.
205. Gennari, C. and Imbimbo, B. (1985). Effects of prednisone and deflazacort on vertebral bone mass. *Calcif. Tissue Int.*, **37**, 592–3.
206. Devogelaer, J. P., Haux, J. P., Dufour, J. P., Esselinckx, W., Stasse, P. and Nagant de Deuxchaisnes, C. (1987). Bone-sparing action of deflazacort versus equipotent doses of prednisone: a double blind study in males with rheumatoid arthritis. In Christiansen, C., Johansen, J. S. and Riis, B. J. (eds), *Osteoporosis 1987* (Copenhagen: Osteopress ApS), pp. 1014–5.
207. Findling, J. W., Adams, N. D., Lemann, J., Gray, R. W., Thomas, C. J. and Tyrell, J. B. (1982). Vitamin D metabolites and parathyroid hormone in Cushing's syndrome: relationship to calcium and phosphorus homeostasis. *J. Clin. Endocrinol. Metab.*, **54**, 1039–44.
208. Van Berkum, F. N. R., Pols, H. A. P., Braun, J. J., Heysteeg, M., Kooij, P. P. M. and Birkenhager, J. C. (1987). Glucocorticoid induced bone loss and treatment with 1α-hydroxyvitamin D_3: a placebo controlled double blind trial. In Christiansen, C., Johansen, J. S. and Riis, B. J. (eds), *Osteoporosis 1987* (Copenhagen: Osteopress ApS), pp. 1033–6.
209. Schwartzman, M. S. and Franck, W. A. (1987). Vitamin D toxicity complicating the treatment of senile, post-menopausal, and glucocorticoid-induced osteoporosis. *Am. J. Med.*, **82**, 224–30.
210. Ringe, J. D., Welzel, D. and Schmid, K. (1987). Therapy of corticosteroid-induced osteoporosis with salmon calcitonin. In Christiansen, C., Johansen, J. S. and Riis, B. J. (eds), *Osteoporosis 1987* (Copenhagen: Osteopress ApS), pp. 1074–6.
211. Reid, I. R., King, A. R., Alexander, C. J. and Ibbertson, H. K. (1988). Prevention of steroid-induced osteoporosis with (3-amino-1-hydroxypropylidene)-1,1-biphosphonate (APD). *Lancet,* **1**, 143–7.
212. Briancon, D. and Meunier, P. J. (1981). Treatment of osteoporosis with fluoride, calcium and vitamin D. *Orthop. Clin. N. Am.*, **12**, 629–48.
213. Gallagher, J. A., Beresford, J. N., McGuire, M. K. B., Ebsworth, N. M., Meats, J. E., Gowen, M., Elford, P., Wright, D., Poser, J., Coulton, L. A., Sharrard,

M., Imbimbo, B., Kanis, J. A. and Russell, R. G. G. (1984). Effects of glucocorticoids and anabolic steroids on cells derived from human skeletal and articular tissues in vitro. *Adv. Exp. Med. Biol.,* **171,** 179–91.

214. Adami, S., Fossaluzza, V., Suppi, R., Constantini, M., Dorizzi, R., Rigolin, F. and Lo Cascio, V. (1987). The low osteocalcin levels of glucocorticoid treated patients can be brought to normal by nandrolone decanoate administration. In Christiansen, C., Johansen, J. S. and Riis, B. J. (eds), *Osteoporosis 1987* (Copenhagen: Osteopress ApS), pp. 1039–40.

215. Reid, D. M., Nicoll, J. J., Smith, M. A., Tothill, P. and Nuki, G. (1987). Treatment of corticosteroid induced osteoporosis: Role of anabolic steroids and microcrystalline calcium hydroxyapatite. In Christiansen, C., Johansen, J. S. and Riis, B. J. (eds), *Osteoporosis 1987* (Copenhagen: Osteopress ApS), pp. 1021–5.

6

THE MANAGEMENT OF OSTEOPOROSIS

R. M. FRANCIS, P. L. SELBY, A. RODGERS and C. E. DAVISON

Osteoporosis is characterized by a reduction in the amount of cortical and trabecular bone in the skeleton, and is associated with an increased risk of fracture. The major osteoporotic fractures are those of the forearm, vertebral body and femoral neck[1], and these cause considerable morbidity and mortality and consume vast health and social service resources[2]. As osteoporosis is difficult, if not impossible, to reverse, the management of the problem should include the prevention of osteoporosis as well as treatment of the established condition.

PREVENTION OF OSTEOPOROSIS

The bone mass at any age, and therefore the risk of fracture, is determined by the peak bone mass, the age at which bone loss begins and the rate at which it proceeds[1]. The prevention of osteoporosis should therefore ideally include the establishment of an optimal peak bone mass, postponement of the onset of bone loss, and reduction of the subsequent rate of bone loss.

The extent to which peak bone mass can be modified is uncertain, and whilst the effects of race, sex and other hereditary factors on bone mass cannot be altered, exercise, dietary calcium intake and hormonal factors may potentially modify the deposition of bone during growth and consolidation.

The importance of exercise in regulating peak bone mass is emphasized by the higher bone mass of athletes than that of more sedentary individuals[3], and the greater bone mass in dominant than non-dominant limbs[4]. Adolescents and young adults should therefore be encouraged to take regular exercise, though females should not exercise to the extent that they become amenorrhoeic, as this may have adverse effects on bone mass because of the associated hypo-oestrogenaemic state[5].

An adequate dietary intake of calcium is also required during childhood and early adult life, to ensure that sufficient calcium is available to be deposited in the skeleton during bone growth and consolidation, though the precise requirement is uncertain. It has been estimated that a dietary intake of 1100 mg calcium is required daily during adolescence, because of a deposition of 300 mg in the skeleton, an obligatory loss of 300 mg calcium daily in the urine and digestive juices, and an efficiency of absorption of only 55%[6]. It is likely that the attainment of a maximal peak bone mass is adversely affected by persistently lower calcium intakes, which are not uncommon in adolescence[7]. Several studies suggest that the dietary calcium intake during bone growth and consolidation influences the peak bone mass[8–10], although the magnitude of this effect is debatable. Children and young adults should therefore be encouraged to eat a balanced diet rich in calcium, and discouraged from excessive dieting because of the association between low body weight and osteoporosis[11]. The major sources of calcium in the diet are dairy products, fish such as sardines and vegetables such as spinach and broccoli. Whilst the consumption of dairy products has become less popular because of their fat content, it should be appreciated that skimmed milk contains slightly more calcium than whole milk with a much lower fat content.

As regards the effects of hormonal factors on peak bone mass, it appears that early menarche, pregnancy and the use of the oral contraceptive pill are associated with a higher bone mass[12], though clearly such measures cannot be advocated in the promotion of an optimal peak bone mass. Nevertheless, secondary amenorrhoea is common in young women[13], and if prolonged may adversely affect bone mass[14]. Amenorrhoea should therefore be considered a potentially serious problem in young women, and investigated and treated as rapidly as possible.

Whilst bone loss appears to start several years before the menopause, it is generally accepted that the menopause is associated with increased bone resorption[15], and an accelerated phase of cortical and trabecular bone loss lasting for up to 10 years[16]. Hormone replacement therapy at the time of the menopause reduces bone resorption[17], prevents both cortical and trabecular bone loss[18], and may substantially reduce the subsequent risk of femoral neck fracture[19]. It is therefore probably the most effective way of delaying the onset of bone loss and reducing the subsequent risk of developing osteoporosis. Unfortunately, there is no consensus as to whether all perimenopausal women should be offered hormone replacement therapy to prevent the development of osteoporosis, or if its use should be targeted on women considered to be most at risk. The risks and benefits of hormone replacement therapy will be discussed later in this chapter, as will possible methods for identifying individuals most at risk of developing osteoporosis.

Whilst hormone replacement therapy may prevent bone loss at the time of the menopause, can anything be done to prevent age-related bone loss subsequently? Metabolic balance studies suggest that the dietary requirement for calcium increases at the menopause from 1 g to 1.5 g daily[20], and as a result postmenopausal women are commonly encouraged to attempt to achieve these calcium intakes. Nevertheless, studies show little or no relationship between dietary calcium intake and the rate of bone loss in women in the years following the menopause[21],[22], suggesting that the dietary intake of calcium is not a major determinant of the rate of bone loss at this time. On the other hand, other studies show an inverse relationship between dietary calcium intake and femoral neck fracture incidence[8,23–25], which may result from an effect of calcium intake on peak bone mass or on the rate of bone loss several decades after the menopause. It would therefore seem prudent to advise that postmenopausal women should have a dietary calcium intake in the region of 1.5 g daily.

Stopping smoking or decreasing tobacco consumption may also potentially reduce the rate of bone loss, as smoking hastens the onset of the menopause[26], depresses circulating oestrogen levels thereafter[27] and possibly inhibits osteoblast function[28]. Alcohol consumption may also have adverse effects on the skeleton at relatively modest intakes[29], and it would seem reasonable to recommend a maximum safe intake of 14 units of alcohol/week for women and 21 units/week for men, as has been advised to protect against other end-organ damage from alcohol consumption.

In view of the apparent benefits of weight-bearing and exercise on the skeleton[30] and the deleterious effects of immobilization[31], people should be encouraged to remain physically active and take regular exercise throughout life. This may protect against bone loss, reduce the risk of falls and improve the overall health of the individual.

The efficiency of calcium absorption from the bowel declines with advancing age[32], and if uncompensated may cause further bone loss (Chapter 3). This reduction in calcium absorption is due to decreased cutaneous production of vitamin D[33], and impaired metabolism to its active metabolite 1,25-dihydroxyvitamin D $(1,25(OH)_2D)$[34]. Ensuring that the elderly are vitamin D replete improves calcium absorption and reduces cortical bone loss[35,36], as well as protecting against the development of osteomalacia. Elderly people should therefore be encouraged to maintain adequate sunlight exposure, and vitamin D supplementation should be considered in housebound and institutionalized individuals.

DETECTION OF ASYMPTOMATIC OSTEOPOROSIS

Osteoporosis is generally considered to be asymptomatic until fractures occur, and because of the potential importance of hormone replacement therapy in preventing further bone loss, much interest has centred on the identification of individuals with early or asymptomatic osteoporosis. The mechanical properties of bone are related to its mineral content, and the risk of fracture is inversely proportional to the bone mass. Investigators have therefore sought methods to measure the bone mass at different sites, and to identify individuals with a low bone mass who may go on to develop osteoporotic fractures. Techniques which have been used to assess bone mass include radiogrammetry, photodensitometry, photon absorptiometry, quantitative computed tomography, ultrasound and quantitative histomorphometry (see Chapter 1). Because of the poor correlation between bone mass at different sites, it appears that in order to detect individuals most at risk of developing vertebral and femoral fractures, techniques which measure bone mass at these sites should be used. Dual-energy X-ray densitometry, dual-photon absorptiometry and quantitative computed tomography are capable of measuring bone mass of the lumbar spine and femoral neck, although these methods differ in precision, radiation exposure and examination time. Whilst these techniques are widely available in the USA, there are few such facilities in the UK, so widespread bone mass screening is impractical at the present time. In addition, there is considerable controversy about the value of such screening techniques[1,37].

An alternative approach is to develop methods which identify women who are losing bone rapidly in the years following the menopause, so that they can be offered hormone replacement therapy. Christiansen has described the use of a combination of body weight, serum alkaline phosphatase and fasting urine calcium/creatinine and hydroxyproline/creatinine to classify women into fast bone losers, slow bone losers and an intermediate group[38]. This may be a useful classification if validated by other groups, although it takes no account of the contribution of bone mass at the menopause to the subsequent risk of developing osteoporosis.

TABLE 6.1   Risk factors for osteoporosis

Caucasian or Asian women
Premature menopause or prolonged amenorrhoea
Positive family history
Short stature, low body weight
Low calcium intake or absorption
Inactivity
Nulliparity
Causes of secondary osteoporosis
Smoking
High alcohol consumption

Adapted from Riggs and Melton[1]

Another method of identifying those at risk of developing osteoporosis is to use historical risk factors (Table 6.1). Unfortunately, these risk factors are not of equal importance, and the appropriate weighting for each has not yet been established[1]. Nevertheless, it may ultimately prove possible to develop a risk factor profile or scoring system, to identify those women likely to have a reduced bone mass. In the meanwhile, it would appear that the risk of developing osteoporosis is related to the number of risk factors present in an individual, so that hormone replacement therapy should be particularly considered in menopausal women with a number of risk factors for osteoporosis[1].

IDENTIFICATION OF ESTABLISHED OSTEOPOROSIS

Osteoporosis is associated with an increased risk of fracture, often occurring after only minimal trauma, and the major osteoporotic fractures are those of the forearm, vertebral body and femoral neck[1]. Fractures of the forearm and femur are generally easy to diagnose, but vertebral crush fractures are more difficult to detect clinically, as some may be asymptomatic and there are many other causes of acute back pain. Typically vertebral crush fractures lead to episodes of acute back pain lasting 6–8 weeks before settling to a more chronic backache. The back pain may be associated with a loss of height of several inches, and there may be evidence of a kyphosis, horizontal skin creases and abdominal protrusion because of the loss of trunk height.

INVESTIGATION OF ESTABLISHED OSTEOPOROSIS

What investigations should be performed in a patient with established osteoporosis? In subjects with forearm fractures, X-rays are performed to confirm the presence of a fracture, and to ascertain its position. The prevalence of secondary osteoporosis is unknown in this group, and further investigation is generally only performed if there is clinical suspicion of an underlying cause of bone loss.

As mentioned above, vertebral crush fractures may be more difficult to diagnose, so spine X-rays should be performed in patients with acute back pain to look for vertebral deformation or the presence of other pathology. Such X-rays may also show lytic or sclerotic lesions, indicating the presence of myeloma or skeletal metastases. Secondary osteoporosis is common in patients with vertebral crush fractures, occurring in 20–35% of women and 40–55% of men[1,39,40]. Identification of secondary osteoporosis is important, as specific treatment of the underlying condition may prevent or reduce further bone loss. It is our usual practice to perform plasma biochemical profile, full blood count, ESR, thyroid function tests and serum and urine immunoelectrophoresis in all osteoporotic patients presenting with vertebral crush fractures, and to measure serum testosterone and gonadotrophins in male patients with spinal osteoporosis. Plasma biochemical profile, full blood count and ESR are usually normal in primary osteoporosis, although there may be a transient elevation in alkaline phosphatase after a fracture. The presence of hypercalcaemia, anaemia or ESR raises the possibility of myeloma or skeletal metastases, and requires further investigation which may include bone marrow examination and isotope bone scan. Thyroid function tests may reveal the presence of previously undetected thyrotoxicosis, and serum testosterone and gonadotrophins may indicate unsuspected hypogonadism in osteoporotic men. Serum and urine immunoelectrophoresis should probably be performed in all patients with vertebral crush fractures, even in the absence of hypercalcaemia, raised ESR or radiological evidence of lytic lesions, as such individuals may still have unrecognized myeloma.

Although femoral neck fracture is an acknowledged complication of osteoporosis, the difference in bone mass between elderly patients with femoral fracture and age-matched control subjects is small, and other factors such as postural stability and frequency of falls appear to be major determinants of the risk of fracture in this age group. Investigations are therefore of limited value in patients with femoral neck fracture, although they may be required on occasions to confirm a diagnosis of secondary osteoporosis or other underlying bone disorders such as osteomalacia or Paget's disease. The prevalence of secondary osteoporosis in patients with femoral neck fracture is unknown. Nevertheless, X-rays of the fractured femur may demonstrate lytic or sclerotic lesions indicating the presence of myeloma or skeletal metastases. Routine full blood count, ESR, plasma biochemical profile and thyroid function tests may also occasionally indicate the possibility of secondary osteoporosis. Paget's disease of the fractured femur will be apparent on X-ray, and usually requires no further investigation. Histological evidence of osteomalacia may be found in a proportion of patients with femoral neck fracture[41], although the diagnosis may not always be apparent. Radiological changes of osteomalacia are present only in the most severe cases, and the biochemical diagnosis of osteomalacia may be difficult in the elderly[42]. Bone biopsy at the time of surgical fixation may therefore be worthwhile in individuals at risk of osteomalacia, because they are housebound or have a past history of anticonvulsant treatment or gastric surgery. Alternatively, it may be argued that all elderly patients with femoral neck fracture are vitamin D deficient and at risk of osteomalacia, and that they should therefore all be routinely treated with oral vitamin D 1000 units daily or intramuscular vitamin D 300 000 units every 6–12 months.

TREATMENT OF ESTABLISHED OSTEOPOROSIS

A number of therapeutic agents have actions on bone and are used in the treatment of osteoporosis. They may be classified into agents which predominantly reduce bone resorption and therefore reduce or prevent further bone loss, and those which stimulate bone formation thereby increasing bone mass. An increase in bone mass may not necessarily be accompanied by a corresponding improvement in the mechanical properties of bone, particularly when the trabecular architecture has been largely disrupted by the osteoporotic process. It should also be appreciated that agents which primarily reduced bone resorption will lead to a later secondary reduction in bone formation, because of the close coupling of the two processes of bone resorption and formation. Antiresorptive agents such as oestrogens and calcitonin may therefore cause a small increase in bone mass, during the transient uncoupling of bone formation and resorption, though this is not sustained in the longer term.

Treatments for osteoporosis need to be taken for long periods of time in order to have a significant effect on bone mass, and many are associated with a variety of side-effects. Which patients with established osteoporosis should therefore be treated? Whilst there is an association between forearm fractures and fractures of the vertebrae and femur, the association is relatively weak, so that this group is not the most appropriate on which to target treatment to prevent bone loss[43]. The association between vertebral crush fractures and femoral fractures is greater than that between forearm and vertebral/femoral fractures[43], so treatment to prevent further bone loss or restore bone mass should be considered in all patients with vertebral crush fractures, in the hope of reducing the risk of further fractures. Treatment to prevent further bone loss is of little value in patients with femoral neck fracture, because of the severity of osteoporosis and the poor life expectancy, and it may be more effective to consider measures to reduce the risk of falls. Treatments which increase bone mass may be more effective, though there is little information on their use in patients with femoral neck fractures.

OESTROGENS

Oestrogen has a profound antiresorptive action on bone cells, and its lack at the time of the menopause is an important cause of bone loss in women (Chapter 4). It is therefore not surprising that oestrogen replacement therapy is one of the major methods of preventing and treating osteoporosis. It must be recalled, however, that oestrogens act on bone to reduce resorption without stimulating bone formation[44], so that whilst oestrogen therapy has an important role in the prevention of postmenopausal bone loss, it is incapable of repairing significant loss once it has occurred. Nevertheless, the initiation of oestrogen treatment is associated with a small increase in bone mass due to the transient uncoupling of one formation and resorption, though the increase is not sustained.

The foregoing should not be taken to imply that oestrogen treatment is without any benefit in patients with established osteoporosis. Since it appears likely that fracture risk will increase as bone mass continues to decline[1,45], any therapy which reduces further bone loss will decrease the risk of subsequent fractures. This has been borne out in those studies which have examined the rate of vertebral fracture incidence in women treated with oestrogen[46,47].

Studies of the effects of oestrogen upon bone have demonstrated a dose–response effect[48], and any therapy aimed at protecting skeletal mass must therefore ensure an adequate dose of oestrogen is administered. The daily dose levels which are necessary are 0.625 mg of conjugated oestrogens (Premarin), 15 μg of ethinyloestradiol, 1–2 mg of micronized oestradiol or oestradiol valerate (Progynova) or 25–50 μg of transdermal oestradiol (Estraderm)[49–52]. Because of the similarity of the dose–response curves for the various aspects of oestrogen's action, it is likely that a dose of oestrogen which is sufficient to relieve a patient's climacteric symptoms will be adequate to protect her skeleton[52]

As well as ensuring that oestrogen is given in a large enough dose, it is important that it be given for a sufficiently long period of time to have a beneficial effect. Case–control studies of oestrogen use in the prevention of femoral neck fracture indicate that a period of treatment of at least 5 years is necessary before any benefit is apparent[19,53]. Although more precise data as to the optimal duration of treatment for the prevention of osteoporosis are not available, it is our practice to recommend that hormone replacement be given for a minimum of 10 years or until the age of 60, whichever occurs later. In a woman who has already sustained an osteoporotic fracture, or in whom there is other evidence of significant bone loss, then such treatment should be indefinite.

In addition to the benefits of oestrogen treatment on the skeleton, it also has a beneficial effect on plasma lipoproteins[54], and on the incidence of cardiovascular and cerebrovascular disease[55]. Whilst this advantageous effect on cardiovascular and cerebrovascular disease may be partly offset by the addition of a cyclical progestogen[56], which is necessary if a woman has an intact uterus (see later), some benefit is still likely.

There are a number of contraindications to the use of oestrogen therapy, including breast or endometrial carcinoma, thromboembolic disease, ischaemic heart disease, cerebrovascular disease, peripheral vascular disease, severe hypertension, migraine and jaundice. We consider a history of breast or endometrial carcinoma an absolute contraindication to oestrogen treatment, whilst the other conditions are relative contraindications. Occasionally we will use oestrogens in a woman with a relative contraindication, providing she understands the increased risks of such treatment and is prepared to accept them.

Oestrogen treatment may be associated with minor side-effects such as nausea, fluid retention, breast tenderness, headache and an increase in blood pressure. These may be related to the oral route of administration and a first-pass effect on hepatic protein synthesis. Such side-effects may potentially be avoided by alternative methods of oestrogen delivery using transdermal patches or implants.

Treatment with oestrogens has also been associated with more serious complications such as thromboembolic disease. Whilst high doses of 'synthetic' oestrogens increase coagulability, it has been argued that the lower dose of the so-called 'natural' oestrogens used for hormone replacement therapy are not associated with an increased risk of thromboembolism[57]. Nevertheless, it is preferable to use an alternative to oestrogen first in patients with a history of thromboembolism, or to administer oestrogen using transdermal patches or implants. This avoids the non-physiological stimulation of the liver which is thought to lead to increased coagulability.

The other side-effect of oestrogen which has aroused concern is an increased risk of cancer. Only two tumours are significantly associated with oestrogen administration – those of the endometrium and breast[58]. Fortunately, the addition of cyclical progestogen to the oestrogen for at least 12 days each month reduces the risk of endometrial hyperplasia to, or even below, that of untreated women[59]. It appears likely that progestogens will also reduce the risk of endometrial cancer, though good epidemiological evidence for this is awaited. Several studies show that the addition of a progestogen does not impair, and might even enhance, the protective effects of oestrogen on bone[60,61]. Unfortunately, this protection is achieved at the expense of a regular monthly withdrawal bleed in the majority of patients, and a significant number of these find this unacceptable and discontinue treatment[62]. Furthermore, most progestogens currently in use diminish the beneficial effects of oestrogen on plasma lipoprotein profiles[56]. Nevertheless, we advise that if a woman has an intact uterus and is to receive oestrogen treatment, she should also be given a progestogen for 12 days each month to protect the endometrium.

In the case of breast cancer the evidence is less clear-cut, but most studies would suggest that there is a very small increase in risk with oestrogen treatment[58]. Although one group has reported that this is reduced by the addition of cyclical progestogens[63], this is not the general view[55]. However, if the increased risk of developing breast cancer is weighed against the beneficial effects of oestrogen upon the skeleton and cardiovascular and cerebrovascular disease, there is an overwhelming positive balance in favour of hormone replacement[64].

Prior to starting hormone replacement therapy we check the blood pressure, examine the breasts and do a cervical smear. During treatment we check the blood pressure and examine the breasts every 6 months, and recommend cervical smear every 3 years. Endometrial biopsy is performed only if irregular or unexpected vaginal bleeding occurs.

Despite the overall benefits of hormone replacement therapy, there remains some resistance to its use amongst British women and their medical advisors. Although this may not hamper the short-term use of hormone treatment for climacteric symptoms, it leads to opposition to its longer-term use in the prevention and treatment of osteoporosis.

PROGESTOGENS

In view of the problems, both real and perceived, relating to the use of oestrogens in postmenopausal women, there is considerable pressure to develop an alternative hormonal treatment for osteoporosis. Several different groups of compounds have been examined with this goal in mind, including progestogens, androgens and anabolic steroids. The uses of androgens and anabolic steroids will be considered later, whilst this section will examine the use of progestational agents in the prevention of bone loss.

In addition to the native hormone progesterone, the progestogens currently available can be separated into two groups: the 17-hydroxyprogesterone derivatives including medroxyprogesterone acetate and megestrol acetate, and the 19-nortestosterone derivatives such as norethisterone, norgestrel and ethinylestrenol. Progesterone, 17-hydroxyprogesterone derivatives and 19-nortestosterone derivatives have all been examined for their ability to reduce postmenopausal bone loss.

An early report suggested that progesterone might inhibit bone resorption *in vitro*[65], but this was at supraphysiological concentrations which were later shown to be toxic[66,67]. A subsequent study was unable to demonstrate any significant reduction in bone resorption when progesterone was administered at physiological levels to postmenopausal women[68].

The evidence concerning the 17-hydroxyprogesterone derivatives is less clear-cut. Whilst very high doses of medroxyprogesterone acetate given either parenterally or orally are capable of reducing bone resorption[69,70], this is not observed when more conventional doses of the drug are given orally[68]. Furthermore, the closely related compound megestrol acetate appears to have only limited action on bone[71].

Most of the work on the effect of progestogens on bone has been performed with the 19-nortestosterone derivatives, and all appear to act on bone. Although there is some controversy in the literature as to whether their action is primarily anabolic or anticatabolic, it seems likely that the 19-nortestosterone derivatives reduce bone resorption rather than stimulate bone formation, in an analogous manner to oestrogens[72]. In addition to short-term biochemical studies two compounds, norethisterone and lynestrol, have been shown to reduce long-term postmenopausal bone loss[73-75]. Longer-term studies of the effect of these agents on fracture incidence are not available.

Since these compounds are derived from testosterone and not oestrogen, they do not possess the same spectrum of side-effects, and so can be used in subjects in whom the use of oestrogen is contraindicated. Some workers have suggested that they are poorly tolerated, but their data relate only to women who are adequately oestrogenized, and not to the use of these agents alone in postmenopausal women. In contrast, we have found that norethisterone in doses of 2.5–5 mg daily is well tolerated in postmenopausal women. An additional benefit is that these compounds do not stimulate endometrial proliferation, and there is accordingly no need for regular withdrawal bleeds. We advise that the norethisterone be taken daily for 3 weeks, after which the therapy is withheld for a week, when any endometrium which has previously been stimulated by endogenous or exogenous oestrogen will be shed. Following this the drug is taken on a daily basis, and any further episodes of bleeding require full gynaecological assessment, as for any other postmenopausal bleeding. We find that norethisterone is an attractive treatment to women who are several years past their menopause but still have an intact uterus, and who do not face the prospect of renewed menstruation with equanimity. Clearly the indications for its use are the same as for oestrogen itself, and the duration of treatment with norethisterone should be the same as if oestrogen were being used.

CALCIUM SUPPLEMENTS

The use of calcium supplements in the prevention and treatment of osteoporosis remains controversial[76]. The rationale for their use is that the majority of individuals take insufficient calcium in the diet to offset the obligatory loss of calcium in the digestive juices and urine, and that calcium is therefore drained from the skeleton to maintain normo-calcaemia[76]. In addition, the efficiency of calcium absorption from the bowel is decreased in osteoporosis[77,78], thereby increasing the dietary requirement for calcium. Nevertheless, as mentioned earlier, there is little or no relationship between dietary calcium intake and rates of bone loss in postmenopausal women[21,22], suggesting that physiological variation in dietary calcium intake is not an important determinant of bone loss. On the other hand, calcium supplements may not serve as simple physiological dietary supplements, but may act pharmacologically by increasing plasma calcium[79], leading to enhanced calcitonin secretion[80], reduction of circulating parathyroid hormone (PTH)[81] and $1,25(OH)_2D[17]$, and decreased bone resorption[82].

The use of calcium supplements containing 1 g elemental calcium daily is associated with biochemical evidence of decreased bone resorption at 1 week, and this appears to be maintained during longer-term treatment[82]. Treatment with calcium supplements containing at least 800 mg elemental calcium reduces the rate of cortical bone loss in normal[18,83–89] and osteoporotic subjects[46,86], although it has no effect on trabecular bone loss[18]. Calcium supplements may also reduce the incidence of further vertebral deformation in patients with established osteoporosis[46,47], but there is little data on the risk of femoral fractures in such patients. Other studies indicate that individuals with a high dietary calcium intake may have a lower risk of femoral neck fracture[8,23–25], but this may be due to an effect on the peak bone mass rather than on the rate of bone loss[8–10].

Calcium supplementation is therefore no substitute for oestrogen therapy, because of the lack of effect on trabecular bone loss, and the smaller reduction in cortical bone loss[18]. It may be useful, however, in patients who are unable or unwilling to take oestrogens because of age, contraindications or side-effects. It has also been suggested that the use of calcium supplements may reduce the dose of oestrogen required to prevent bone loss, but these data have been challenged, and further confirmatory studies are awaited[87].

There are a number of calcium supplements available in the UK, including effervescent calcium lactate gluconate (Sandocal; each tablet containing 400 mg elemental calcium), microcrystalline hydroxyapatite compound (Ossopan; each tablet containing 176 mg elemental calcium) and chewable calcium carbonate (Calcichew; each tablet containing 500 mg elemental calcium). Whilst differences in bioavailability have been reported with these preparations[81], there is little evidence that any supplement is more effective in the treatment of primary osteoporosis, although one paper suggests that microcrystalline hydroxyapatite compound is more effective than calcium lactate gluconate in preventing bone loss in primary biliary cirrhosis[88]. The choice of calcium supplement should probably be determined by cost and individual tolerability, but it is important to give sufficient calcium to suppress bone resorption and reduce cortical bone loss. We therefore generally give supplements containing 1000–1200 mg elemental calcium daily. Calcium supplements are usually well tolerated, and can be given indefinitely, but should be avoided in patients with hypercalcaemia, moderate to severe renal impairment and renal stone disease.

VITAMIN D AND VITAMIN D METABOLITES

Although physiological doses of vitamin D (500–1000 units daily) may reduce cortical bone loss in the elderly[36] and prevent the development of osteomalacia, such treatment has no role in the management of established osteoporosis. Calcium absorption is lower in osteoporotic individuals than in age-matched normal subjects[39,77,78], though it is unclear if this results from an intrinsic defect in the absorption mechanism[89], or from low plasma $1,25(OH)_2D$ concentrations due either to a failure of the renal 1α-hydroxylase enzyme to respond to PTH[90] or to suppression of PTH production by increased bone resorption[91]. Physiological doses of vitamin D have little or no effect on calcium absorption in osteoporosis, and high doses (10 000–40 000 units daily) are required to overcome the malabsorption of calcium[78]. Despite the improvement in calcium absorption, high-dose vitamin D treatment does not reduce and may accelerate bone loss[46], possibly by the stimu-

159

lation of bone resorption by supraphysiological 25-hydroxyvitamin D concentrations.

Early studies with the vitamin D metabolites calcitriol and alfacalcidol in doses of 1–2 μg daily also showed improvement in calcium absorption[92,93] though no beneficial effect on bone loss was observed[46], possibly because of stimulation of bone resorption by high plasma 1,25(OH)$_2$D levels[94]. More recent work has shown low-dose calcitriol and alfacalcidol (0.25–0.5 μg daily) can increase calcium absorption in osteoporotic subjects[95–97], with little increase in plasma 1,25(OH)$_2$D[95,97]. This is associated with biochemical evidence of decreased bone resorption[96,97] which, if sustained, may reduce the rate of bone loss. Nevertheless, the use of vitamin D metabolites in osteoporosis is still experimental, and cannot be generally recommended.

TESTOSTERONE AND ANABOLIC STEROIDS

Testosterone is as important for the integrity of the male skeleton as oestrogen is for the female, as hypogonadism is a well-established cause of bone loss in men as in women[98,99]. In hypogonadal men administration of testosterone appears to increase bone mass by stimulating bone formation[99]. It is our practice to administer 100–250 mg of testosterone esters (Sustanon) fortnightly by intramuscular injection to such patients, to render them clinically and biochemically eugonadal. The effect of the newer oral testosterone preparations such as testosterone undecanoate (Restandol) upon bone mass in these patients is yet to be determined, but one would expect them to be as effective as the parenteral depot preparations, as long as the patient is rendered eugonadal. The use of testosterone in male osteoporotic patients with normal gonadal function is still under assessment, and cannot yet be recommended generally.

Administration of testosterone to women with osteoporosis might be expected to lead to unacceptable side-effects, but it has been used as an adjunct to subcutaneous oestrogen pellets by at least one group without such problems[100]. This group has recently reported an increase in bone mass in a group of women treated in this fashion[100], suggesting that androgens given in an appropriate manner may benefit women with osteoporosis.

Anabolic steroids have been used for treatment of osteoporosis in men and women, and both orally administered stanozolol (Stromba) and intramuscular nandrolone decanoate (Decadurabolin) have been shown to increase bone mass[101,102], presumably by stimulating bone formation. It is possible that these compounds have an additional effect on bone resorption, as they also reduce the urinary excretion of hydroxyproline, suggesting that they decrease collagen breakdown[103]. Unfortunately, both these drugs have significant androgenic side-effects, and whilst this is of little consequence when they are used in men, it makes them unacceptable to many women. In addition, there are considerable doubts about their long-term safety, with abnormalities of liver function and even hepatocellular tumours being reported[104]. In the light of this it is impossible to recommend their widespread general use for the treatment of osteoporosis, although they may be of use in patients who have proved resistant to other therapies. Such a therapeutic decision should probably be taken at a specialist centre.

CALCITONIN

Calcitonin is the hypocalcaemic hormone secreted by the C cells of the thyroid in response to an increase in plasma calcium, which inhibits bone resorption by a rapid decrease in osteoclast activity and a later effect on osteoclast recruitment[105,106]. Whilst calcitonin is a potent inhibitor of bone resorption *in vitro*, its physiological role in the regulation of bone resorption and calcium homeostasis is uncertain. Plasma calcitonin levels are generally lower in women than in men[107,108], and may fall with advancing age[109,110], though this is not a universal finding[107]. It has also been suggested that a relative deficiency of calcitonin may be involved in the pathogenesis of osteoporosis[111], though longstanding calcitonin deficiency is not associated with a reduced bone mass[112]. Calcitonin should therefore be considered a pharmacological antiresorptive agent rather than a physiological replacement therapy.

Calcitonin is commercially available in porcine and salmon forms, and these are more potent than human calcitonin. The hormone is usually administered subcutaneously, and may cause side-effects such as nausea, vomiting and facial flushing. An intra-nasal preparation has recently been developed, which is well tolerated with a reported reduction in adverse effects, though this is not yet commercially available[113].

Clinical studies on the use of calcitonin in osteoporosis have produced variable results, and are therefore difficult to interpret. There is a shortage of well-controlled, long-term studies, and little or no information is available on the effects of treatment on fracture rates. Calcitonin increases PTH by its hypocalcaemic effects, so most studies have used calcitonin together with calcium or vitamin D supplements, to diminish PTH secretion and any secondary increase in bone resorption. Early work showed that calcium and vitamin D supplements were effective in preventing the expected increase in PTH with calcitonin therapy, though no benefit was apparent on bone mass measured histologically[114]. Subsequent studies showed that calcitonin treatment could prevent bone loss, and even lead to a small increase in bone mass, probably because of the transient uncoupling of bone resorption and formation. Gennari compared a control group given calcium alone to two other groups given 100 units of calcitonin either on alternate days or daily. After 1 year there appeared to be a dose-dependent increase in vertebral bone mineral content with rises of 4% and 8.5% respectively in the treatment groups[115]. These results were confirmed by Mazzuoli using alternate-day calcitonin and measuring radial bone mineral content[116]. Chesnut compared a control group receiving calcium and vitamin D supplements with a group also treated with calcitonin, and demonstrated an increase in total-body calcium after 18 months in the group receiving calcitonin, though this beneficial effect appeared to be declining after 26 months[117].

The problem of apparent resistance to prolonged calcitonin therapy is well recognized[113,118], though suggestions that this is due to antibody formation or down-regulation of the receptors may not be the explanation. Indeed studies confirming the presence of antibodies have shown that their appearance does not correlate with the efficacy of calcitonin, and the time scale of their formation does not correspond to the development of resistance[117].

In conclusion, there is some evidence that daily or alternate-day treatment with calcitonin can decrease bone resorption and present bone loss. No information is available regarding the effects of treatment on fracture, the most important consequence of osteoporosis. The drug is expensive, and is usually given parenterally, though some benefits are claimed for the intra-nasal route. Overall, it probably has no advantages over other therapies, though it may be useful where other treatments cannot be used. Calcitonin also acts as a centrally acting analgesic, and so may occasionally be useful in the presence of severe back pain due to vertebral crush fractures, though other analgesics may be easier to use and are considerably cheaper.

FLUORIDE

It has been appreciated for several decades that individuals living in areas with a high fluoride content in water (>4 ppm) have a higher bone mass and lower fracture incidence than individuals from low-fluoride areas[119–121]. Fluoride was first used in the treatment of osteoporosis in 1961 by Rich and Ensinck, who demonstrated an increase in calcium retention[122]. Subsequent studies showed that fluoride treatment improved calcium balance, stimulated bone formation and increased trabecular bone mass.

Fluoride is rapidly absorbed after oral administration with almost 100% bioavailability if taken in the fasting state, though absorption is diminished by food, especially when this contains calcium[123]. The serum concentration in those not taking fluoride is usually about 1 μmol/l and a therapeutic range of 5–15 μmol/l has been suggested[124]. Plasma levels are, however, not readily available, and are very variable due to a half-life of only 4 hours. Up to 60% of absorbed fluoride accumulates in bone and the remainder is excreted by the kidneys[124]. Secretion and reabsorption of fluoride also occurs in the kidneys, so care must be exercised in the therapeutic use of fluoride in patients with renal impairment[124]. Fluoride attaches to apatite in bone in preference to hydroxyl groups, and the resulting fluoroapatite crystals are more resistant to resorption than hydroxyapatite[124]. Osteoblastic activity is also stimulated, leading to an increase in osteoid production and trabecular bone volume, though the mechanism of this remains unclear[124]. Calcium and vitamin D supplements are necessary to allow mineralization of the osteoid to proceed, and thus prevent the development of osteomalacia[125].

The normal remodelling cycle for bone is up to a year, and this is prolonged by fluoride treatment to 2–4 years. Fluoride will therefore not produce obvious benefit immediately, and any benefit may continue after cessation of treatment[126]. It has also been suggested that intermittent therapy could be used, with 6 months treatment followed by 6 months without, to allow mineralization to occur[127]. However, the benefits may still be occurring at 5 years, and longer periods of treatment may therefore be better. Any assessment of the efficacy of any fluoride regime has to consider the long latent period before benefit occurs, but many studies have been relatively short-term (1–2 years), and definite conclusions cannot be drawn.

Problems with fluoride treatment are common. About 25% of patients fail to respond to fluoride treatment, though these cannot be identified prior to treatment[128]. Adverse effects occur in up to 50% of those treated, and include dyspepsia, peptic ulceration and articular and periarticular changes producing joint pain and swelling[129]. Gastrointestinal effects can be reduced by using slow-release preparations. Occasionally fluoride has a direct toxic effect on osteoblasts leading to osteomalacia, and this may occur with moderate doses, and after only short periods of treatment. It appears to be independent of calcium and vitamin D status, and is reversible if fluoride is stopped. It is recommended that the dose of sodium fluoride is 40–80 mg daily, with lower doses proving ineffective. High doses increase trabecular bone mass, though cortical bone mass is unchanged or diminished. Indeed, as total body calcium does not appear to increase, it is likely that increased vertebral bone mass may be at the expense of the appendicular skeleton[130]. The new bone may also not be of normal quality, and the increased bone mass may not correlate with increased strength[131]. Although resistance to compressive forces increases, resistance to torsional strain is less[132]. The only true measure of success of any treatment regime is reduction of fracture rate, and consistent results with fluoride are lacking, with some studies showing a reduction and others an apparent increase[47,133].

In conclusion, fluoride administration is capable of increasing bone mass, though the effect is delayed, and bone strength may not be improved. Many patients will not respond and others will suffer adverse effects. Further research is therefore necessary to select the right patients and the most useful regime before fluoride should be considered an established therapy for osteoporosis.

BISPHOSPHONATES

Pyrophosphate is a naturally occurring substance found in plasma, urine, saliva and synovial fluid which inhibits crystallization of calcium phosphate from solution, slows the transformation of amorphous calcium phosphate into crystals, inhibits the aggregation of crystals into large clusters and prevents the dissolution of hydroxyapatite crystals[134]. Bisphosphonates are synthetic analogues of pyrophosphate, in which a P–C–P bond replaces the P–O–P bond of pyrophosphate. The P–C–P bonds are stable to heat, chemical agents and enzymatic hydrolysis, and remain in bone until released during bone resorption[134]. Intestinal absorption of these compounds is low (1–10%) and very variable. The half-life in plasma is only a few minutes, with 50% localizing to bone and the remainder being excreted in the urine unchanged. Bisphosphonates are powerful inhibitors of crystallization and soft tissue calcification, but in contrast to pyrophosphate, they also inhibit bone resorption[134].

Although the reduction in bone resorption seen with bisphosphonates may in part be due to inhibition of crystal dissolution, it is likely that they also affect osteoclast number and function. Bisphosphonates may inhibit osteoclast recruitment, alter osteoclast morphology, reduce lactic acid production, inhibit lysosomal enzymes and decrease prostaglandin synthesis[135]. There is no correlation between their *in vitro* and *in vivo* effects, and the mechanism of action may differ from compound to compound. Nevertheless, as bisphosphonates are bound in the skeleton and are taken up by osteoclasts during bone resorption, their action may persist for a long period after administration has ceased.

Bisphosphonates are well tolerated and have a low toxicity. High doses given intravenously can lead to complex formation and a temporary fall in ionized calcium. Prolonged administration of 1-hydroxyethylidene–1,1-bisphosphonate (EHDP, disodium etidronate) leads to inhibition of mineralization with accumulation of osteoid.

Chronic treatment with EHDP or dichloromethylenebisphosphonate (Cl_2MBP) may markedly decrease bone turnover, leading to increased fragility and fractures. Other bisphosphonates have produced changes in the lungs and digestive mucosa, and higher doses have been shown to produce renal lesions, thymic atrophy and immunological changes.

Clinical studies on the use of bisphosphonates have suffered from the same problems as other proposed therapies, in that they are poorly controlled, have no long-term follow-up and little information on fracture rates. Early studies using continuous treatment with high-dose EHDP demonstrated no benefit. Jowsey et al.[136] showed an increase in osteoid after 3 months treatment with oral EHDP 10–20 mg/kg per day, and this appeared to be dose-related. Heaney and Saville[137] demonstrated a marked decrease in bone resorption after 6–12 months treatment with oral EHDP 20 mg/kg per day, though this was matched by an equally large decrease in mineralization, with no apparent overall benefit. More recent studies have used bisphosphonates intermittently and as part of coherence therapy (see later). Anderson used 15 days treatment with EHDP, preceded by phosphate for 3 days, and followed by 72 days on no therapy[138]. Cycles were repeated every 90 days, and led to large increases in trabecular bone volume of 50–160%. However, an increase in osteoid was again seen, suggesting that the increase in bone mass may not be accompanied by an increase in bone strength. Alternative bisphosphonates with less effect on mineralization may produce more worthwhile results, and studies using 3-amino-1-hydroxypropylidene-1,1-bisphosphonate (APD) have shown appreciable increases in bone mineral content of spine and appendicular skeleton. Following on Anderson's work, other groups have tried cyclical bisphosphonate regimes. Storm reported an increase in spine bone mass of $6 \pm 1.9\%$ after eight cycles of 15 weeks (2 weeks EHDP 400 mg/day, 13 weeks off) compared to a fall of $5.2 \pm 2.4\%$ on placebo[139]. These results have been confirmed in a study by Genant et al., who demonstrated no increase in radial bone, but no loss either[140]. Miller et al. used phosphate followed by EHDP to produce a highly significant increase in spine bone mass[141], but Mallette and LeBlanc, using higher dose short pulses of EHDP, produced variable results[142]. Whilst the results of treatment with bisphosphonates look promising, further studies are needed to determine the best regime, in particular which bisphosphonate to use, in what dose, and for how long.

THIAZIDES

Thiazides are well known to reduce urinary calcium excretion, and it has been shown that elderly individuals taking thiazides have a lower risk of femoral fracture[143]. A study of hypertensive men using hydro-chlorthiazide also showed an increase in bone mass at several sites when compared with hypertensives not on thiazides, or to normo-tensive subjects[144]. However, further studies have been unable to confirm this beneficial effect and Transbøl et al. failed to show any persistent effect on bone loss in women after 2 years[145]. Therefore, although useful in improving calcium balance, evidence is lacking to support the use of thiazides in the treatment of osteoporosis.

PARATHYROID HORMONE

The effects of PTH have been studied in small numbers of patients with osteoporosis. Reeve et al. found that daily injections of PTH increased trabecular bone volume[146], though there was no improve-ment in calcium balance, and cortical bone mass may decrease[147]. It therefore seems likely that the improvement in trabecular bone is at the expense of cortical bone, though studies are proceeding to establish if the adverse effects on cortical bone mass can be avoided by the concomitant administration of an anti-resorptive agent. PTH should therefore be considered an investigational drug in the treatment of osteoporosis for the time being.

COHERENCE THERAPY

The work of Frost on the microanatomy of bone suggested that its turnover was determined by the activity of separate discrete groups of bone-resorbing and bone-forming cells acting in concert, in what he termed a basic multicellular unit (BMU). Thus he suggested that all bone remodelling consisted of a period of bone resorption lasting some 2–3 weeks, followed after an apparent resting or reversal phase by a much longer period of formation[148]. This theory predicts that any bone formation must be preceded by an episode of resorption. If the skeletal mass is constant, the amount of bone laid down by each BMU will exactly replace the amount removed in the earlier resorptive phase. In patients with osteoporosis there is a slight shortfall within each BMU, which eventually leads to the observed decrease in bone mass.

Frost postulated that if it were possible to find an agent that would minimize the amount of bone resorbed by each BMU without affecting the bone laid down by the forming phase, it might be possible to alter this balance in favour of bone formation and ultimately lead to an increased bone mass. In order to achieve this it is necessary to get as many BMUs as possible at the same stage in their cycle. To do this an agent such as PTH, phosphate or fluoride is given to *activate* as many BMUs as possible to start resorbing, following this an anti-resorptive agent such as calcitonin or a bisphosphonate is administered to *depress* the resorptive process. After that the therapy is withdrawn to *free* bone formation to proceed normally. Finally, in order to build up a significant bone mass it is necessary to *repeat* the cycle on several occasions. Because the various BMUs are all brought into phase in the course of this therapy it is frequently referred to as 'coherence therapy' or alternatively as ADFR (Activate–Depress–Free–Repeat)[149].

A variety of different ADFR regimes have been proposed, and at present none can be generally recommended. Initial studies examining one regimen's effect by bone biopsy looked very promising[138], but more recent work with a different protocol showed no benefit in terms of bone mass measured absorptiometrically[150]. In view of this discrepancy, such treatments should be considered only as part of a clinical trial at the present time.

EXERCISE

As mentioned earlier, weight-bearing and regular exercise may affect trabecular bone architecture by stimulating osteoblastic new bone formation, although the exact mechanism remains unknown. Regular exercise may allow the attainment of an optimal peak bone mass[3,4], reverse the bone loss seen after immobilization[31] and inhibit involutional bone loss[30]. A number of prospective studies have examined the effects of different exercise programmes on bone mass, with conflicting results[151], although the overall conclusion is that physical activity may inhibit further bone loss and perhaps even increase bone mass. Unfortunately, these studies have been criticized for inadequate sample size, lack of randomization of subjects to treatment and control groups, and failure to take into account other variables such as medications, diet or additional exercise. Despite these reservations, it is generally recommended that osteoporotic subjects take regular physical exercise. The exercise programme should be tailored to the individual's age, previous activity and any concomitant disease such as ischaemic heart disease. Regular weight-bearing exercise – particularly brisk walking, light running, social dancing and group aerobics – appears the most useful. Swimming is less effective for strengthening the bone as it is non-weight-bearing, but may be useful in established osteoporosis when it may reduce muscle spasm and pain associated with a recent vertebral crush fracture. Other benefits of regular exercise include improvement of general physical performance, the overall feeling of well-being, reduction of the risk of falls and the opportunity for social interaction.

OTHER MEASURES

In addition to considering treatment in established osteoporosis, measures should be taken to reduce the risk of falls. These should include the removal of environmental hazards such as loose-fitting carpets, the treatment of underlying physical conditions and the avoidance of drugs which increase the risk of falls.

REFERENCES

1. Riggs, B. L. and Melton, L. J. III (1986). Involutional osteoporosis. *N. Engl. J. Med.*, **314**, 1676–86.

2. Wallace, W. A. (1987). The scale and financial importance of osteoporosis. *Int. Med.,* Suppl. 12, 3–4.
3. Nilson, B. E. and Westlin, N. E. (1971). Bone density in athletes. *Clin. Orthop.,* **77,** 179–82.
4. Jones, H. H., Priest, J. D., Hayes, W. C., Tichenor, C. C. and Nagel, D. A. (1977). Humeral hypertrophy in response to exercise. *J. Bone. Jt. Surg.,* **59A,** 204–8.
5. Drinkwater, B. L., Nilson, K., Chesnut, C. H. III, Bremner, W. J., Shainholtz, S. and Southworth, M. B. (1984). Bone mineral content of amenorrheic and eumenorrheic athletes. *N. Engl. J. Med.,* **311,** 277–81.
6. Robinson, C. J. (1987). The importance of calcium intake in preventing osteoporosis. *Int. Med.,* Suppl. 12, 28–9.
7. Hackett, A. F., Rugg-Gunn, A. J., Allinson, M., Robinson, C. J., Appleton, D. R. and Eastoe, J. E. (1984). The importance of fortification of flour with calcium and the sources of Ca in the diet of 375 English adolescents. *Br. J. Nutr.,* **51,** 193–7.
8. Matkovic, V., Kostial, K., Simonovic, I., Buzina, R., Brodarec, A. and Nordin, B. E. C. (1979). Bone status and fracture rates in two regions of Yugoslavia. *Am. J. Clin. Nutr.,* **32,** 540–9.
9. Sandler, R. B., Slemenda, C. W., LaPorte, R. E., Cauley, J. A., Schramm, M. M., Barresi, M. L. and Kriska, A. M. (1985). Postmenopausal bone density and milk consumption in childhood and adolescence. *Am. J. Clin. Nutr.,* **42,** 270–4.
10. Kanders, B., Dempster, D. W. and Lindsay R. (1988). Interaction of calcium nutrition and physical activity on bone mass in young women. *J. Bone. Min. Res.,* **3,** 145–9.
11. Saville, P. D. and Nilsson, B. E. R. (1966). Height and weight in symptomatic postmenopausal osteoporosis. *Clin. Orthop.,* **45,** 49–54.
12. Goldsmith, N. F. and Johnston, J. O. (1975). Bone mineral: effects of oral contraceptives, pregnancy and lactation. *J. Bone J. Surg.,* **57A,** 657–68
13. Bachmann, G. A. and Kemmann, E. (1982). Prevalence of oligomenorrhea and amenorrhea in a college population. *Am. J. Obstet. Gynecol.,* **144,** 98–102
14. Cann, C. E., Martin, M. C., Genant, H. K. and Jaffe, R. B. (1984). Decreased spinal mineral content in amenorrheic women. *J. Am. Med. Assoc.,* **251,** 626–9.
15. Hodgkinson, A. and Thompson, T. (1982). Measurement of the fasting urine hydroxyproline:creatinine ratio in normal adults and its variation with age and sex. *J. Clin. Pathol.,* **35,** 807–11.
16. Aitken, J. M., Hart, D. M., Anderson, J. B., Lindsay, R., Smith, D. A. and Speirs, C. F. (1973). Osteoporosis after oophorectomy for non-malignant disease in premenopausal women. *Br. Med. J.,* **2,** 325–8.
17. Nordin, B. E. C., Peacock, M., Aaron, J. E., Crilly, R. G., Heyburn, P. J., Horsman, A. and Marshall, D. H. (1980). Osteoporosis and osteomalacia. *Clin. Endocrinol. Metab.,* **9,** 177–205.
18. Riis, B., Thomsen, K. and Christiansen, C. (1987). Does calcium supplementation prevent postmenopausal bone loss? A double blind controlled study. *N. Engl. J. Med.,* **316,** 173–7.
19. Kiel, D. P., Felson, D. T., Anderson, J. J., Wilson, P. W. F. and Moskovitz, M. A. (1987). Hip fractures and the use of estrogen in postmenopausal women. *N. Engl. J. Med.,* **317,** 1169–74.
20. Heaney, R. P., Recker, R. R. and Saville, P. D. (1978). Menopausal changes in

calcium balance performance. *J. Lab. Clin. Med.,* **92,** 953–63.

21. Riggs, B. L., Wahner, H. W., Melton, L. J. III, Richelson, L. S., Judd, H. L. and O'Fallon, W. M. (1987). Dietary calcium intake and rates of bone loss in women. *J. Clin. Invest.,* **80,** 979–82.
22. Stevenson, J. C., Whitehead, M. I., Padwick, M., Endacott, J. A., Sutton, C., Banks, L. M., Freemantle, C., Spinks, T. J. and Hesp, R. (1988). Dietary intake of calcium and postmenopausal bone loss. *Br. Med. J.,* **297,** 15–17.
23. Holbrook, T. L., Barrett-Connor, E. and Wingard, D. L. (1988). Dietary calcium and risk of hip fracture: 14-year prospective population study. *Lancet,* **2,** 1046–9.
24. Cooper, C., Barker, D. J. P. and Wickham, C. (1988). Physical activity, muscle strength, and calcium intake in fracture of the proximal femur in Britain. *Br. Med. J.,* **297,** 1443–6.
25. Lau, E., Donnan, S., Barker, D. J. P. and Cooper, C. (1988). Physical activity and calcium intake in fracture of the proximal femur in Hong Kong. *Br. Med. J.,* **297,** 1441–3.
26. Jick, H., Porter, J. and Morrison, A. S. (1977). Relation between smoking and the age of natural menopause. *Lancet,* **1,** 1354–5.
27. Jensen, J., Christiansen, C. and Rødbro, P. (1985). Cigarette smoking, serum estrogens and bone loss during hormone-replacement therapy early after menopause. *N. Engl. J. Med.,* **313,** 973–5.
28. De Vernejoul, M. C., Bielakoff, J., Herve, M., Gueris, J., Hott, M., Modrowski, D., Kuntz, D., Miravet, L. and Ryckewaert, A. (1983). Evidence for defective osteoblastic function. A role for alcohol and tobacco consumption in osteoporosis in middle-aged men. *Clin. Orthop.,* **179,** 107–15.
29. Nordin, B. E. C. and Polley, K. J. (1987). Metabolic consequences of the menopause. *Calcif. Tissue Int.,* **41,** (Suppl. 1), 1–59.
30. Krølner, B., Toft, B., Pors Nielsen, S. and Tøndevold, E. (1983). Physical exercise as prophylaxis against involutional bone loss: a controlled trial. *Clin. Sci.,* **64,** 541–6.
31. Krølner, B. and Toft, B. (1983). Vertebral bone loss: an unheeded effect of therapeutic bed rest. *Clin. Sci.,* **64,** 537–40.
32. Bullamore, J. R., Gallagher, J. C., Wilkinson, R., Nordin, B. E. C. and Marshall, D. H. (1970). Effect of age on calcium absorption. *Lancet,* **2,** 535–7.
33. Baker, M. R., Peacock, M. and Nordin, B. E. C. (1980). The decline in vitamin D status with age. *Age Ageing,* **9,** 249–52.
34. Francis, R. M., Peacock, M. and Barkworth, S. A. (1984). Renal impairment and its effects on calcium metabolism in elderly women. *Age Ageing,* **13,** 14–20.
35. Francis, R. M., Peacock, M., Storer, J. H., Davies, A. E. J., Brown, W. B. and Nordin, B. E. C. (1983). Calcium malabsorption in the elderly: the effect of treatment with oral 25-hydroxyvitamin D_3. *Eur. J. Clin. Invest.,* **13,** 391–6.
36. Nordin, B. E. C., Baker, M. R., Horsman, A. and Peacock, M. (1985). A prospective trial of the effect of vitamin D supplementation on metacarpal bone loss in elderly women. *Am. J. Clin. Nutr.,* **42,** 470–4.
37. Hall, F. M., Davis, M. A. and Baran, D. T. (1987). Bone mineral screening for osteoporosis. *N. Engl. J. Med.,* **316,** 212–14.
38. Christiansen, C., Riis, B. J. and Rødbro, P. (1987). Prediction of rapid bone loss in postmenopausal women. *Lancet,* **1,** 1105–8.
39. Francis, R. M., Peacock, M., Marshall, D. H., Horsman, A. and Aaron, J. E.

(1989). Spinal osteoporosis in men. *Bone Mineral*, **5**, 347–57.

40. Peacock, M., Francis, R. M. and Selby, P. L. (1983). Vitamin D and osteoporosis. In Dixon, A. St J., Russell, R. G. G. and Stamp, T. C. B. (eds), *Osteoporosis: Multidisciplinary Problem* (London: Academic Press), pp. 245–54.

41. Aaron, J. E., Gallagher, J. C., Anderson, J., Stasiak, L., Longton, E. B., Nordin, B. E. C. and Nicholson, M. (1974). Frequency of osteomalacia and osteoporosis in fractures of the proximal femur. *Lancet*, **1**, 229–33.

42. Campbell, G. A., Hosking, D. J., Kemm, J. R. and Boyd, R. V. (1986). Timing of screening for osteomalacia in the acutely ill elderly. *Age Ageing*, **15**, 156–63.

43. Marshall, D. H., Horsman, A., Simpson, M., Francis, R. M. and Peacock, M. (1984). Fractures in elderly women: prevalence of wrist, spine and femur fractures and their concurrence. In Christiansen, C., Arnaud, C. D., Nordin, B. E. C., Parfitt, A. M., Peck, W. A. and Riggs, B. L. (eds), *Osteoporosis* (Glostrup, Denmark: Glostrup Hospital), pp. 361–3.

44. Lafferty, F. W., Spencer, G. E. Jr and Pearson, O. H. (1964). Effects of androgens, estrogens and high calcium intakes on bone formation and resorption in osteoporosis. *Am. J. Med.*, **36**, 514–28.

45. Riggs, B. L., Wahner, H. W., Dunn, W. L., Mazess, R. B., Offord, K. P. and Melton, L. J. III (1981). Differential changes in bone mineral density of the appendicular and axial skeleton with aging. Relationship to spinal osteoporosis. *J. Clin. Invest.*, **67**, 328–35.

46. Nordin, B. E. C., Horsman, A., Crilly, R. G., Marshall, D. H. and Simpson, M. (1980). Treatment of spinal osteoporosis in postmenopausal women. *Br. Med. J.*, **280**, 451–4.

47. Riggs, B. L., Seeman, E., Hodgson, S. F., Taves, D. R. and O'Fallon, W. M. (1982). Effect of the fluoride/calcium regimen on vertebral fracture occurrence in postmenopausal osteoporosis: comparison with conventional therapy. *N. Engl. J. Med.*, **306**, 446–50.

48. Horsman, A., Jones, M., Francis, R. and Nordin, C. (1983). The effect of estrogen dose on postmenopausal bone loss. *N. Engl. J. Med.*, **309**, 1405–7.

49. Geola, F. L., Frumar, A. L., Tataryn, I. V., Lu, K. H., Hershman J. M., Eggena, P., Sambhi, M. P. and Judd, H. L. (1980). Biological effects of various doses of conjugated estrogens in postmenopausal women. *J. Clin. Endocrinol. Metab.*, **51**, 620–5.

50. Mandel, F. P., Geola, F. L., Lu, J. K. H., Eggena, P., Sambhi, M. P., Hershman, J. M. and Judd, H. L. (1982). Biologic effects of various doses of ethinyl estradiol in postmenopausal women. *Obstet. Gynecol.*, **59**, 673–9.

51. Jones, M. M., Pearlman, B., Marshall, D. H., Crilly, R. G. and Nordin, B. E. C. (1982). Dose-dependent response of FSH, flushes and urinary calcium to estrogen. *Maturitas*, **4**, 285–90.

52. Selby, P. L. and Peacock, M. (1986). The dose dependent response of symptoms, pituitary and bone to transdermal oestrogen in postmenopausal women. *Br. Med. J.*, **293**, 1337–9.

53. Weiss, N. S., Ure, C. L., Ballard, J. H., Williams, A. R. and Darling, J. R. (1980). Decreased risk of fracture of the hip and lower forearm with postmenopausal use of estrogen. *N. Engl. J. Med.*, **303**, 1195–8.

54. Wahl, P. W., Warnick, G. R. and Albers, J. J. (1981). Distribution of lipoproteins, triglycerides and lipoprotein cholesterol in an adult population by age, sex and hormone use. *Atherosclerosis*, **39**, 111–24.

55. Hunt, K. and Vessey, M. P. (1987). Long term effects of hormone replacement therapy. *Br. J. Hosp. Med.,* **38,** 450–60.
56. Hirvonen, E., Malkonen, M. and Manninen, V. (1981). Effects of different progestogens on lipoproteins during postmenopausal replacement therapy. *N. Engl. J. Med.,* **304,** 560–3.
57. Campbell, S. and Whitehead, M. I. (1981). Potency and hepatocellular effects of oestrogen after oral, percutaneous and subcutaneous administration. In van Keep, P. (ed.), *The Controversial Climacteric* (Lancaster: MTP Press), 103–25.
58. Hunt, K., Vessey, M., McPherson, K. and Coleman, M. (1987). Long term surveillance of mortality and cancer incidence in women receiving hormone replacement therapy. *Br. J. Obstet. Gynaecol.,* **94,** 620–35.
59. Whitehead, M. I., Townsend, P. T. and Pryse-Davies, J. (1981). Effects of estrogens and progestins on the biochemistry and morphology of the postmenopausal endometrium. *N. Engl. J. Med.,* **305,** 1599–605.
60. Crilly, R. G., Marshall, D. H. and Nordin, B. E. C. (1978). The effect of oestradiol valerate/DL norgestrel on calcium metabolism. *Postgrad. Med. J.,* **54,** (Suppl. 2), 47–9.
61. Christiansen, C., Riis, B. J., Nilas, L., Rødbro, P. and Deftos L. (1985). Uncoupling of bone formation and resorption by combined oestrogen and progestogen therapy in postmenopausal osteoporosis. *Lancet,* **2,** 800–1.
62. Jones, M. M., Francis, R. M. and Nordin, B. E. C. (1982). Five year follow up of oestrogen therapy in 94 women. *Maturitas,* **4,** 123–30.
63. Gambrell, R. D., Maier, R. C. and Sanders B. T. (1983). Decreased incidence of breast carcinoma in post menopausal estrogen-progestogen users. *Obstet. Gynecol.,* **62,** 435–43.
64. Hillner, B. E., Hollenberg, H. P. and Pauker S. G. (1986). Postmenopausal estrogen in prevention of osteoporosis: benefit virtually without risk if cardiovascular effects are considered. *Am. J. Med.,* **80,** 1115–27.
65. Atkins, D. and Peacock, M. (1975). A comparison of the effects of the calcitonins, sex steroids and thyroid hormones on the response of bone to parathyroid hormone in tissue culture. *J. Endocrinol.,* **64,** 573–83.
66. Caputo, C. B., Meadows, D. and Raisz, L. G. (1976). Failure of estrogens and androgens to inhibit bone resorption in tissue culture. *Endocrinology,* **98,** 1065–8.
67. Francis, R. M., Peacock, M., Taylor, G. A., Kahn, A. J. and Teitelbaum, S. L. (1985). How do oestrogens modulate bone resorption? In Norman, A. W., Schaefer, K., Grigoleit, H.-G. and Herrath, D. v. (eds), *Vitamin D: Chemical, Biochemical and Clinical Update* (Berlin, New York: Walter de Gruyter), pp. 479–80.
68. Selby, P. L. (1989). Studies of the action of sex steroids on bone in the postmenopausal women. M.D. dissertation. (Cambridge: University of Cambridge), pp. 80–91.
69. Lobo, R. A., McCormick, W., Singer, F. and Roy, S. (1984). Depomedroxyprogesterone acetate compared with conjugated estrogen for the treatment of postmenopausal women. *Obstet. Gynecol.,* **63,** 1–5.
70. Franchi, M., La Fianza, A., Dore, R., Babilonti, L. and Bolis, P. F. (1987). Effects of progestins on bone density of postmenopausal patients with endometrial carcinoma. In Christiansen, C., Johansen, J. S. and Riis, B. J. (eds), *Osteoporosis 1987* (Copenhagen: Osteopress ApS), pp. 979–80.

173

71. Erlik, Y., Meldrum, D. R. and Lagasse, L. D. (1981). Effect of megestrol acetate on flushing and bone metabolism in postmenopausal women. *Maturitas*, **3**, 167–72.

72. Selby, P. L., Peacock, M., Barkworth, S. A., Brown, W. B. and Taylor, G. A. (1985). Early effects of ethinyloestradiol and norethisterone treatment on bone resorption and calcium regulating hormones. *Clin. Sci.*, **69**, 265–71.

73. Dequeker J. and De Muylder, E. (1982). Long-term progestogen treatment and bone remodelling in peri-menopausal women: a longitudinal study. *Maturitas*, **4**, 309–13.

74. Abdalla, H. I., Hart, D. M., Lindsay, R., Leggate, I. and Hooke, A. (1986). Prevention of bone mineral loss in postmenopausal women by norethisterone. *Obstet. Gynecol.*, **66**, 789–92.

75. Selby, P. L., Horsman, A. and Peacock, M. (1987). Norethisterone as an alternative to oestrogen in the management of postmenopausal osteoporosis. In Christiansen, C., Johansen, J. S. and Riis, B. J. (eds), *Osteoporosis 1987* (Copenhagen: Osteopress ApS), pp. 555–6.

76. Francis, R. M. (1989). The calcium controversy. *Journal of the Royal College of Physicians of London* (In press).

77. Gallagher, J. C., Riggs, B. L., Eisman, J., Hamstra, A., Arnaud, S. B. and De Luca, H. F. (1979). Intestinal calcium absorption and serum vitamin D metabolites in normal subjects and osteoporotic patients. Effect of age and dietary calcium. *J. Clin. Invest.*, **64**, 729–36.

78. Gallagher, J. C., Aaron, J., Horsman, A., Marshall, D. H., Wilkinson, R. and Nordin, B. E. C. (1973). The crush fracture syndrome in postmenopausal women. *Clin. Endocrinol. Metab.*, **2**, 293–315.

79. Horowitz, M., Morris, H. A., Hartley, T. F., Need, A. G., Wishart, J., Ryan, P. and Nordin, B. E. C. (1987). The effect of an oral calcium load on plasma ionized calcium and parathyroid hormone concentrations in osteoporotic postmenopausal women. *Calcif. Tissue Int.*, **40**, 133–6.

80. Beringer, T. O., Ardill, J. and Taggart, H. M. (1986). Effect of calcium and stanozolol on calcitonin in patients with femoral fracture. *Bone Mineral*, **1**, 289–95.

81. Reid, I. R., Hannan, S. F., Schooler, B. A. and Ibbertson, H. K. (1986). The acute biochemical effects of four proprietary calcium preparations. *Aust. N.Z. J. Med.*, **16**, 193–7.

82. Horowitz, M., Need, A. G., Philcox, J. C. and Nordin, B. E. C. (1985). The effect of calcium supplements on plasma alkaline phosphatase and urinary hydroxyproline in postmenopausal women. *Horm. Metab. Res.*, **17**, 311–12.

83. Recker, R. R., Saville, P. D. and Heaney, R. P. (1977). Effect of estrogens and calcium carbonate on bone loss in postmenopausal women. *Ann. Intern. Med.*, **87**, 649–55.

84. Horsman, A., Gallagher, J. C., Simpson, M. and Nordin, B. E. C. (1977). Prospective trial of oestrogen and calcium in postmenopausal women. *Br. Med. J.*, **2**, 789–92.

85. Albanese, A. A., Edelson, A. H., Lorenze, E. J., Woodhull, M. L. and Wein, E. H. (1975). Problems of bone health in the elderly: ten year study. *N.Y. State J. Med.*, **75**, 326–36.

86. Smith, D. A., Anderson, J. J. B., Aitken, J. M. and Shimmins, J. (1975). The effects of calcium supplements of the diet on bone mass measurements. In

Kuhlencordt, F. and Kruse, H. P. (eds), *Calcium Metabolism, Bone and Metabolic Bone Disease* (Berlin: Springer), pp. 278–82.

87. Ettinger, B., Genant, H. K. and Cann, C. E. (1987). Postmenopausal bone loss is prevented by treatment with low-dose estrogen with calcium. *Ann. Intern. Med.*, **106**, 40–5.

88. Epstein, O., Kato, Y., Dick, R. and Sherlock, S. (1982). Vitamin D, hydroxyapatite and calcium gluconate in treatment of cortical bone thinning in postmenopausal women with primary biliary cirrhosis. *Am. J. Clin. Nutr.*, **36**, 426–30.

89. Francis, R. M., Peacock, M., Taylor, G. A., Storer, J. H. and Nordin, B. E. C. (1984). Calcium malabsorption in elderly women with vertebral fractures: evidence for resistance to the action of vitamin D metabolites on the bowel. *Clin. Sci.*, **66**, 103–7.

90. Slovik, D. M., Adams, J. S., Neer, R. M., Holick, M. F. and Potts, J. T. Jr. (1981). Deficient production of 1,25-dihydroxyvitamin D in elderly osteoporotic patients. *N. Engl. J. Med.*, **305**, 372–4.

91. Riggs, B. L., Hamstra, A. and De Luca, H. F. (1981). Assessment of 25-hydroxyvitamin D 1α hydroxylase reserve in postmenopausal osteoporosis by administration of parathyroid extract. *J. Clin. Endocrinol. Metab.*, **53**, 833–5.

92. Lindholm, T. S., Sevastikoglou, J. A. and Lindgren, U. (1977). Treatment of patients with senile, postmenopausal and corticosteroid-induced osteoporosis with 1α-hydroxyvitamin D_3 and calcium: short- and long-term effects. *Clin. Endocrinol.*, **7** (Suppl.), 183–9.

93. Gallagher, J. C., Jerpbak, C. M., Jee, W. S. S., Johnston, K. A., De Luca, H. F. and Riggs, B. L. (1982). Administration of 1,25-dihydroxyvitamin D_3 to patients with postmenopausal osteoporosis: short- and long-term effects on bone and calcium metabolism. *Proc. Nat. Acad. Sci.*, **79**, 3325–9.

94. Maierhofer, W. J., Gray, R. W., Cheung, H. S. and Lemann, J. Jr. (1983). Bone resorption stimulated by elevated serum $1,25(OH)_2$ vitamin D concentrations in healthy men. *Kidney Int.*, **24**, 555–60.

95. Francis, R. M. and Peacock, M. (1987). Local action of oral 1,25-dihydroxycholecalciferol on calcium absorption in osteoporosis. *Am. J. Clin. Nutr.*, **46**, 315–18.

96. Nordin, B. E. C., Need, A. G., Morris, H. A. and Horowitz, M. (1988). The rationale for calcitriol therapy in osteoporosis. In Norman, A. W., Schafer, K., Grigoleit, H.-G. and Herrath, D. v. (eds), *Vitamin D: Molecular, Cellular and Clinical Endocrinology* (Berlin, New York: Walter de Gruyter), pp. 826–35.

97. Francis, R. M., Robinson, C. J., Davison, C. E. and Rodgers, A. The short term effects of alfacalcidol in elderly osteoporotic women. In Norman, A. W., Schaefer, K., Grigoleit, H.-G. and Herrath, D. v. (eds), *Vitamin D: Molecular Cellular and Clinical Endocrinology* (Berlin, New York: Walter de Gruyter), pp. 846–7.

98. Seeman, E., Melton, L. J. III, O'Fallon, W. M. and Riggs, B. L. (1983). Risk factors for spinal osteoporosis in men. *Am. J. Med.*, **75**, 977–83.

99. Francis, R. M., Peacock, M., Aaron, J. E., Selby, P. L., Taylor, G. A., Thompson, J., Marshall, D. H. and Horsman, A. (1986). Osteoporosis in hypogonadal men: role of decreased plasma 1,25-dihydroxyvitamin D, calcium malabsorption, and low bone formation. *Bone,* **7**, 261–8.

100. Savvas, M., Studd, J. W. W., Fogelman, I., Dooley, M., Montgomery, J. and

Murby, B. (1988). Skeletal effects of oral oestrogen compared with subcutaneous oestrogen and testosterone in postmenopausal women. *Br. Med. J.,* **297,** 331–3.

101. Chesnut, C. H., Ivey, J. L., Gruber, H. E., Matthews, M., Nelp, W. B., Sisom, K. and Baylink, D. J. (1983). Stanozolol in postmenopausal osteoporosis: therapeutic efficacy and possible mechanisms of action. *Metabolism,* **29,** 559–62.

102. Need, A. G., Chatterton, B. E., Walker, C. J., Steurer, T. A., Horowitz, M. and Nordin, B. E. C. (1986). Comparison of calcium, calcitriol, ovarian hormones and nandrolone in the treatment of osteoporosis. *Maturitas,* **8,** 275–80.

103. Yates, A. J. P., Gray, R. E. S., Percival, R. C., Galloway, J. H., Russell, R. G. G. and Kanis, J. A. (1984). Skeletal effects of stanozolol in osteoporosis. In Christiansen, C., Arnaud, C. D., Nordin, B. E. C, Parfitt, A. M., Peck, W. A. and Riggs, B. L. (eds), *Osteoporosis* (Glostrup, Denmark: Glostrup Hospital), pp. 509–11.

104. Davis, M. and Williams, R. (1985). Hepatic disorders. In Davies, D. M. (ed.), *Textbook of Adverse Drug Reactions* (Oxford: Oxford University Press), pp. 250–90.

105. Friedman, J. and Raisz, L. G. (1965). Thyrocalcitonin, inhibitor of bone resorption in tissue culture. *Science,* **150,** 1465–7.

106. Aliapoulios, M. A., Goldhaber, P. and Munson, P. L. (1966). Thyrocalcitonin inhibition of bone resorption induced by parathyroid hormone in tissue culture. *Science,* **151,** 330–1.

107. Body, J.-J. and Heath, H. III (1983). Estimates of circulating monomeric calcitonin: physiological studies in normal and thyroidectomized man. *J. Clin. Endocrinol. Metab.,* **57,** 897–903.

108. Stevenson, J. C. (1982). Regulation of calcitonin and parathyroid hormone secretion by oestrogens. *Maturitas,* **4,** 1–7.

109. Deftos, L. J., Weisman, M. H., Williams, G. W., Karpf, D. B., Frumar, A. M., Davidson, B. J., Parthemore, J. G. and Judd, H. L. (1980). Influence of age and sex on plasma calcitonin in human beings. *N. Engl. J. Med.,* **302,** 1351–3.

110. Shamonki, I. M., Frumar, A. M., Tataryn, I. V., Meldrum, D. R., Davidson, B. H., Parthemore, J. G., Judd, H. L. and Deftos, L. J. (1980). Age-related changes of calcitonin secretion in females. *J. Clin. Endocrinol. Metab.,* **50,** 437–9.

111. Taggart, H. M., Chesnut, C. H. III, Ivey, J. L., Baylink, D. J., Sisom, K., Huber, M. B. and Roos, B. A. (1982). Deficient calcitonin response to calcium stimulation in postmenopausal osteoporosis? *Lancet,* **1,** 475–8.

112. Hurley, D. L., Tiegs, R. D., Wahner, H. W. and Heath, H. III. (1987). Axial and appendicular bone mineral density in patients with long-term deficiency or excess calcitonin. *N. Engl. J. Med.,* **317,** 537–41.

113. Reginster, J. Y., Denis, D., Albert, A., Deroisy, R., Lecart, M. P., Fontaine, M. A., Lambelin, P. and Franchimont, P. (1987). 1-Year controlled randomised trial of prevention of early postmenopausal bone loss by intranasal calcitonin. *Lancet,* **2,** 1481–3.

114. Jowsey, J., Riggs, B. L., Kelly, P. J. and Hoffman, D. L. (1978). Calcium and salmon calcitonin in treatment of osteoporosis. *J. Clin. Endocrinol. Metab.,* **47,** 633–9.

115. Gennari, C., Chierichetti, S. M., Bigazzi, S., Fusi, L., Gonnelli, S., Ferrara, R. and Zacchei, F. (1985). Comparative effects on bone mineral content of calcium

and calcium plus salmon calcitonin given in two different regimens in post-menopausal osteoporosis. *Curr. Ther. Res., 38*, 455–64.

116. Mazzuoli, G. F., Passeri, M., Gennari, C., Minisola, S., Antonelli, R., Valtorta, C., Palummeri, E., Cervellin, G. F., Gonnelli, S. and Francini, G. (1986). Effects of salmon calcitonin in postmenopausal osteoporosis: a controlled double-blind clinical study. *Calcif. Tissue Int., 38*, 3–8.

117. Gruber, H. E., Ivey, J. L., Baylink, D. J., Matthews, M., Nelp, W. B., Sisom, K. and Chesnut, C. H. III (1984) Long-term calcitonin therapy in postmenopausal osteoporosis. *Metabolism, 33*, 295–303.

118. Aloia, J. F., Vaswani, A., Kapoor, A., Yeh, J. K. and Cohn, S. H. (1985). Treatment of osteoporosis with calcitonin, with and without growth hormone. *Metabolism, 34*, 124–9.

119. Bernstein, D. S., Sadowsky, N., Hegsted, D. M., Guri, C. D. and Stave, F. J. (1966). Prevalence of osteoporosis in high- and low-fluoride areas in North Dakota. *J. Am. Med. Assoc., 198*, 499–504.

120. Alffram, P. A., Hernborg, J. and Nilsson, B. E. R. (1969). The influence of a high fluoride content in the drinking water on the bone mineral mass in man. *Acta Orthop. Scand., 40*, 137–42.

121. Simonen, O. and Laitinen, O. (1985). Does fluoridation of drinking-water prevent bone fragility and osteoporosis? *Lancet, 2*, 432–3.

122. Rich, C. and Ensink, F. (1961). Effect of sodium fluoride on calcium metabolism of human beings. *Nature, 191*, 184–5.

123. Frey, H. (1986). Fluoride in the treatment of osteoporosis. *Acta Med. Scand., 220*, 193–4.

124. Kanis, J. A. and Meunier, P. J. Should we use fluoride to treat osteoporosis?: a review. *Q. J. Med., 53*, 145–64.

125. Jowsey, J., Riggs, B. L., Kelly, P. J. and Hoffman, D. L. (1972). Effect of combined therapy with sodium fluoride, vitamin D and calcium in osteoporosis. *Am. J. Med., 53*, 43–9.

126. Harrison, J. E., McNeill, K. G., Sturtridge, W. C., Bayley, T. A., Murray, T. M., Williams, C., Tam, C. and Fornasier, V. (1981). Three-year changes in bone mineral mass of postmenopausal osteoporotic patients based on neutron activation analysis of the central third of the skeleton. *J. Clin. Endocrinol. Metab., 52*, 751–8.

127. Kleerkoper, M., Crouch, M., Frame, B., Matthews, C., Matkovic, V., Oliver, I., Rao, D. and Parfitt, A. M. (1979). Effect of sodium fluoride alone on iliac bone remodelling dynamics in osteoporosis. *Calcif. Tissue Int., 28*, 158.

128. Briancon, D. and Meunier, P. J. (1981). Treatment of osteoporosis with fluoride, calcium, and vitamin D. *Orthop. Clin. North Am., 12*, 629–48.

129. Riggs, B. L., Hodgson, S. F., Hoffman, D. L., Kelly, P. J., Johnson, K. A. and Taves, D. (1980). Treatment of primary osteoporosis with fluoride and calcium. Clinical tolerance and fracture occurrence. *J. Am. Med. Assoc., 243*, 446–9.

130. Franke, J., Runge, H., and Fengler, F. (1977). Endemic and industrial fluorosis. In Courvoisier, B., Donath, A. and Baud, C. A. (eds), *Fluoride and Bone* (Bern, Stuttgart, Vienna: Hans Huber), pp. 129–43.

131. Wolinsky, I., Simkin, A. and Guggenheim, K. (1972). Effect of fluoride on metabolism and mechanical properties of rat bone. *Am. J. Physiol., 223*, 46–50.

132. Franke, J., Runge, H., Gray, P., Fengler, F., Wanka, A. and Rempel, H. (1976).

Physical properties of fluorosis bone. *Acta Orthop. Scand., 47,* 20–7.

133. Hedlund, L. R. and Gallagher, J. C. (1989). Increased incidence of hip fracture in osteoporotic women treated with sodium fluoride. *J. Bone Min. Res., 4,* 223–5.

134. Fleisch, H. (1981). Diphosphonates: history and mechanisms of action. *Metab. Bone Dis. Rel. Res., 4/5,* 279–88.

135. Marrs-Simon, P. A., Parent, L. S. and Simkover, R. A. (1988). Use of etidronate disodium in osteoporosis. *Drug Intell. Clin. Pharm., 22,* 239–40.

136. Jowsey, J., Riggs, B. L., Kelly, P. J., Hoffman, D. L. and Bordier, P. (1971). The treatment of osteoporosis with disodium ethane-1-hydroxy-1,1-diphosphonate. *J. Lab. Clin. Med., 78,* 574–84.

137. Heaney, R. P. and Saville, P. D. (1976). Etidronate disodium in postmenopausal osteoporosis. *Clin. Pharmacol. Ther., 20,* 593–604.

138. Anderson, C., Cape, R. D. T., Crilly, R. G., Hodsman, A. B. and Wolfe, B. M. (1984). Preliminary observations of a form of coherence therapy for osteoporosis. *Calcif. Tissue Int., 36,* 341–3.

139. Storm, T., Thamsborg, G., Sørensen, O. H. and Lund, B. (1987). The effects of etidronate therapy in postmenopausal osteoporotic women: preliminary results. In Christiansen, C., Johansen, J. S. and Riis, B. J. (eds), *Osteoporosis 1987* (Copenhagen: Osteopress ApS), pp. 1172–6.

140. Genant, H. K., Harris, S. T., Steiger, P., Davey, P. F. and Block, J. E. (1987). The effect of etidronate therapy in postmenopausal osteoporotic women: preliminary results. In Christiansen, C., Johansen, J. S. and Riis, B. J. (eds), *Osteoporosis 1987* (Copenhagen: Osteopress ApS), pp. 1177–81.

141. Miller, P. D., Neal, B. J., McIntyre, D. O., Yanover, M. J. and Kowalski, L. (1987). The effect of coherence (ADFR) therapy with phosphate and etidronate on axial bone mineral density in postmenopausal osteoporosis. In Christiansen, C., Johansen, J. S. and Riis, B. J. (eds), *Osteoporosis 1987* (Copenhagen: Osteopress ApS), pp. 884–5.

142. Mallette, L. E. and LeBlanc, A. D. (1987). Cyclic therapy of osteoporosis: use of a brief, high-dose pulse of etidronate as a terminator of osteoclast activity. In Christiansen, C., Johansen, J. S. and Riis, B. J. (eds), *Osteoporosis 1987* (Copenhagen: Osteopress ApS), pp. 944–6.

143. Ray, W. A., Griffin, M. R., Downey, W. and Melton, L. J. III (1989). Long-term use of thiazide diuretics and risk of hip fracture. *Lancet, 1,* 687–90.

144. Wasnich, R. D., Benfante, R. J., Yano, K., Heilbrun, L. and Vogel, J. M. (1983). Thiazide effect on the mineral content of bone. *N. Engl. J. Med., 309,* 344–7.

145. Transbøl, I., Christensen, G. F., Jensen, G. F., Christiansen, C. and McNair, P. (1982). Thiazide for the postponement of postmenopausal bone loss. *Metabolism, 31,* 383–6.

146. Reeve, J., Meunier, P. J., Parsons, J. A., Bernat, M., Bijvoet, O. L. M. and Courpron, P. (1980). Anabolic effect of human parathyroid hormone fragment on trabecular bone in involutional osteoporosis: a multicentre trial. *Br. Med. J., 280,* 1340–4.

147. Hesp, R., Hulme, P., Williams, D. and Reeve, J. (1981). The relationship between changes in femoral bone density and calcium balance in patients with involutional osteoporosis treated with human parathyroid hormone fragment (hPTH 1–34). *Metab. Bone Dis. Rel. Res., 2,* 331–4.

148. Frost, H. M. (1973). *Bone Remodelling and its Relationship to Metabolic Bone Diseases* (Springfield, Illinois: C. C. Thomas).
149. Frost, H. M. (1981). Coherence treatment of osteoporosis. *Orthop. Clin. N. Am.,* **12,** 649–69.
150. Pacifici, R., McMurty, C., Vered, I., Rupich, R. and Avioli, L. V. (1988). Coherence therapy does not prevent axial bone loss in osteoporotic women. *J. Clin. Endocrinol. Metab.,* **66,** 747–53.
151. Martin, A. D. and Houston, C. S. (1987). Osteoporosis, calcium and physical activity. *Can. Med. Assoc. J.,* **136,** 587–93.

INDEX